HEALTH YOUR SELF

DR NIC GILL is a professional strength and conditioning coach and an Associate Professor in Health, Sport and Human Performance. He is best known for his work in rugby, with 18 years working in the sport. Nic has been the strength and conditioning coach for the All Blacks since 2008, a period of unprecedented international success for the team that has included over 150 test match wins and World Cup titles in 2011 and 2015.

Beyond rugby, Nic has experience in a variety of other sports, including work as strength and power coach for the record-breaking rowers Eric Murray and Hamish Bond, and strength and conditioning coach of the New Zealand Track Cycling Endurance team leading up to the 2016 Rio Olympics.

In addition to helping individuals and teams strive towards high performance, Nic is a lifestyle and fitness coach for a number of international corporate organisations and individuals who take their own health, fitness, wellbeing and performance seriously.

Nic continues to study and research many areas of human performance at the University of Waikato, constantly refining and evolving his philosophy for being fit and healthy, and having the winning edge in life and in competition.

www.nicgill.com

SUE PAGE has a PhD from the University of Kent and spent the first part of her working life as a research scientist in New Zealand, England and the Netherlands. In later years she moved from lab bench to office desk, first working as an editor in the book publishing industry, then as a science writer and educator in the agricultural industry. At home, she brings science to the kitchen, creating healthy and delicious vegetarian meals, and totally indulgent cakes and desserts. A keen runner, she has completed many half-marathons, one 100-km run, and several team triathlons and cycling events.

DR NIC GILL
WITH SUE PAGE, PHD

HEALTH YOUR SELF

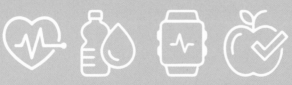

The one-stop handbook to a
healthier, more energetic you

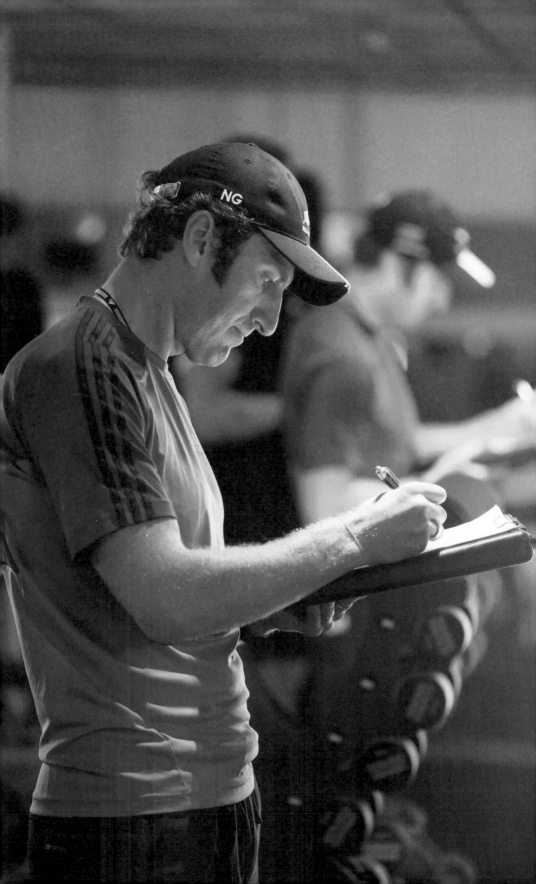

CONTENTS

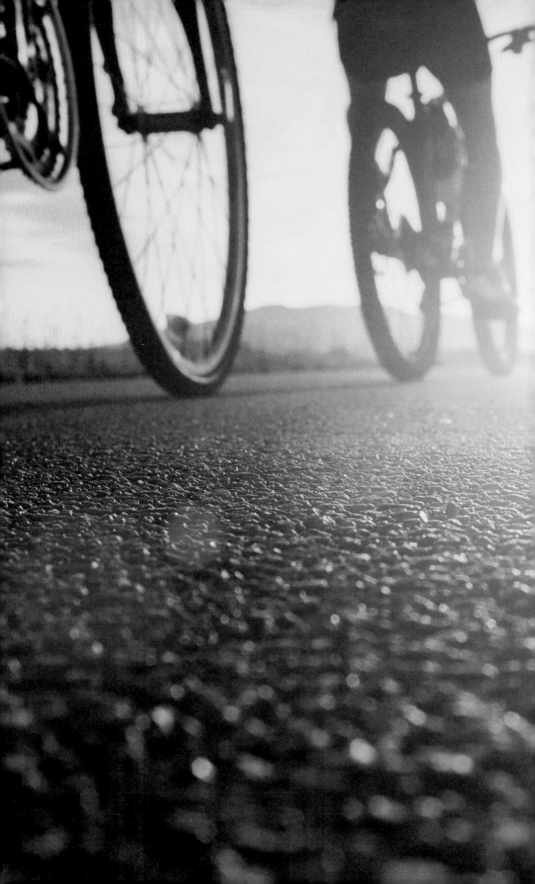

PART ONE

—

THE INSIDE STORY

When it comes to health and fitness, each of us has our own story to tell. As an individual, what you do, feel and value is unique to you, shaped by your genes, environment and experience. The trouble is, those same factors that shape you can also limit you — unless you push your beliefs, stretch your mind and challenge your body, you might never know what else you are capable of achieving. Don't let who you are today limit who you could be tomorrow.

#1
FIT–FAT FLIP-FLOP

I was at university when I first realised I wasn't healthy. I was way out of shape. While I wasn't exactly a candidate for *The Biggest Loser*, I *was* definitely bigger than I'd ever been. About 20 kilograms bigger, in fact. And I was studying physical education . . . I really should have known better.

Up until then, I'd never been unfit or overweight. I grew up in a typical Kiwi family, with barbecues and parties and lots of good food. I never thought about what I ate, and my parents certainly never talked about nutrition. Food was just food – delicious and filling and there for eating.

As a teenager, I was really active. I'd ride my bike for hours on end, then come home and eat a mountain of bread rolls and fresh fruit. I was lean, I was fit. I had no idea that this would change. At age 17 I moved to Dunedin and embraced the lifestyle of a university student. I was still exercising, sure, but I was also spending a lot of time sitting down. I'd changed what I was doing but I hadn't changed how I was eating. And, eventually, it caught up with me.

Weight gain is sneaky. It's so gradual that you usually don't realise what's happening – until one day your clothes don't fit any more, or you find yourself out of breath after climbing a flight of stairs. I'd been at university for about a year and a half when I suddenly found that my rugby shorts were tight around my quads, and not because I'd put on lots of muscle. It was fat. And it wasn't just my shorts: my jeans were tight, my T-shirts were tight – and not in a good way.

I didn't feel good about being overweight, and running was harder than it should have been. So, I started watching what I was eating and exercising more, and gradually I felt better. I was healthier and I had more energy to do the things I loved. My life was back on track, or so I thought.

After I finished my degree at Otago University, I moved to Australia to do a PhD. Along with the study came time at the beach – and Aussie beaches are all about the body. Sun's out, guns out. It made me so much more aware of my body and also of what I was eating. I had an advantage – I was still young, I was into sports and activity, and I was working in the field of exercise and nutrition. But then I got married. Suddenly, life was very different. Back in New Zealand, I got a job as a lecturer and my wife and I started a family. I was tired; my wife was tired. Neither of us was good in the kitchen. Our lives were disorganised, and we were both stressed. Dinner became whatever was easy, something that could be slammed in the oven with no thought or effort. I often sat down to a kilo of chips, three or four sausages and a heap of peas – nutrition didn't come into it.

Not surprisingly, I started to put on weight again. I was struggling to find the time to exercise, I was chronically tired and I was eating rubbish. It would have been a miracle if I *hadn't* gained weight and lost health!

Like all new parents, we battled through and eventually things changed. Our girls grew older, and we got more sleep and had more time to do activities as a family. At the same time, my career was evolving and I started to do research into the connection between nutrition and sports performance. Today there's a lot of awareness of this at an elite sports level, but back then it was a new field. We were all learning as we were going along.

Despite working in this area, I still wasn't as healthy as I would have liked. I knew all about the theory of good nutrition – but that didn't stop me eating when I wasn't hungry, or having a few beers on a regular basis, or eating chocolate every day. These habits were keeping me from being my best, and I wasn't even conscious of that fact.

Things started to change when I read a book that talked about the 'ideal' way to eat. It was based on the idea that ancient warriors only ate once a day, and this helped keep them lean and strong. I decided that it was worth trying – but just for two weeks! It wasn't an easy two weeks, but I'd committed to it so just had to push through it. And I learnt something. I learnt that a lot of the time, my desire to eat is all in my head. I eat breakfast because it's morning. I eat lunch because that's what everyone else at work is doing. I eat dinner with my family because it's a nice social thing to do. I'm not always hungry when I eat – but I eat anyway.

This was a real turning point for me. I hadn't found a magic diet or 'the one true way' of eating. Instead, I'd woken up to what *I* did, to how *I* behaved, to how *my* habits – conscious or not – influenced *my* weight, *my* fitness and *my* health.

I started to experiment with what I ate, when I ate and how much I ate. I'd add a food to my diet, and see how it made me feel. I'd remove something, and see what effect that had. An experiment might last for a few days or a few months – depending on what I was trying to find out. It didn't take me long to discover that a big feed of fish and chips and four beers for dinner on Friday meant that I struggled to feel good through my long run on Saturday. It took a lot longer to see the effect of cutting out my habitual savoury muffin with my mid-morning coffee.

Over time, I developed an approach that worked for me. It's one that still lets me indulge in my favourite foods (chocolate, peanut butter and cheese are high on the list), *and* lets me have a beer or two every now and then, but also one that helps me stay fit, healthy and energised. I use the same principles to help my clients develop their own strategies for optimising their diet, health and lifestyle. It's an approach that can work for anyone who's willing to experiment. And it's not just for professional athletes – a lot of my clients are mums and dads who face those real-life stresses of family, finances and not enough time in the day! What they all have in common is that they know their health matters – and they want to do something about it.

CHANGES AT THE CUTTING EDGE

When I was lecturing at Waikato Institute of Technology (Wintec), I wanted to maintain my connection with sport so volunteered to help out with the Waikato rugby team. I'd spend four hours a week with the guys, putting them through their paces in the gym. The results must have been noticed, because after a while I was asked to work with the Chiefs, which meant that I had a new squad of professional rugby players to look after.

I'd had a brief stint with the All Blacks in 2004; then, in 2008, I became their strength and conditioning coach. This gave me a fantastic opportunity to work with some top-level athletes whose total focus is on being the best they can. If we're on tour, a typical day starts at 7.30 am with a training session that's focused on the game – it's all about the team and what they are trying to achieve. This is the coach's domain. I'm just there as part of the wider training group, keeping an eye out for ways in which individuals could improve. After lunch – and a power nap if I'm lucky – it's my turn to work with the group, and we hit the gym from 2.30 pm until around 6. Here each player has his own plan that he's working to – it's about personalised strength and conditioning for that individual.

When I first started doing this type of work, the individual wasn't considered that important. The thinking at the time was that the players in each position needed to be a certain shape, weight and size - if you were a prop, you were big and heavy and shorter than a lock; if you were anywhere on the back line, you were lighter and faster and no one really cared how tall you were. Strength and conditioning goals were all about getting players to a target weight for their position, about getting them to bench-press or leg-press a specific weight or run 100 metres within a certain time.

Today, that's all changed. There are no pre-existing weight targets or strength targets or speed targets for each position. Instead, we look at the whole person and calculate where we should invest our energy to get the biggest impact. We are now taking a much more holistic view. It's about having fit and healthy athletes - not just muscle monsters who can bash into each other on the field but then fall apart if they get a cold! Strength and conditioning includes taking care of your nutrition (the All Blacks have a full-time dietitian on the team), your sleep (we expect players to aim for 10 hours of sleep a night - and get at least nine), your mobility and your flexibility, as well as your training load.

The principles outlined in this book are exactly the same as the ones that I use with the All Blacks. The focus is not on strength or weight, but on being a fit and healthy individual – that's a recipe for long-term success, no matter what you want out of life.

#2 WHY YOUR HEALTH MATTERS

Most of us are lucky enough to be born with an amazing gift – health. As kids, we take it for granted: running around, eating whatever we like – never thinking that our world might change. As we get older, most of us continue to ignore our health; we have way too many other priorities. Then, one day, we suddenly realise that our health has got up and walked out the door!

This is when we discover that we're a bit bigger than we'd like, or that we can't walk as far as we should be able to, or that our sleep isn't very good. We might find that our thinking's fuzzy, that we've got no energy, that life feels too hard. We can find ourselves suffering from one minor ailment after another, or ending up on three or four medications just to try to stay 'healthy'. Of course, a good diet and lifestyle can't *totally* protect you against any of these outcomes – there are lots of different factors at play – but they *can* help.

SUPERSIZED STATS

\# 1 in 3 New Zealand adults is obese.
\# In 2014–2015 there were around 250,000 overweight or obese children in New Zealand.
\# Only one-third of Australian adults has a healthy bodyweight.
\# Obesity reduces your life expectancy by more than 9 years.
\# In 2016, there were 1.9 billion overweight adults in the world.

OBESITY . . .

increases your risk for depression and anxiety
increases your risk of 'lifestyle' diseases
reduces life quality
reduces life expectancy.

One of the biggest reasons why health matters is that good health lets you enjoy life more! You've been given this one chance to live – why not make the most of it? The better your health, the more you can get out of every day.

If you're a parent, there's another reason why health matters: what you do today, your kids will do in the future. If you can arm yourself with workable strategies to keep yourself and your family healthy, then you'll be able to pass that knowledge on to your kids – and they will have a much better chance of living a long and healthy life as a result.

In general, as we get healthier we become more energised, more confident, more productive. Healthier people are happier people – and who wouldn't want that?

#3 WHAT DOES GOOD HEALTH MEAN TO YOU?

We're all different, and we each have our own idea of what good health is. There's no right or wrong when it comes to this – the main thing is to identify what's important to you and then work towards that. Here are some examples of what good health might mean to different people:

Being able to run a marathon.
Being able to run around with the kids.
Being able to climb Mount Kilimanjaro.
Being able to climb two flights of stairs without puffing.
Being able to see your six-pack abs.
Being able to see your feet.
Waking up feeling energised.
Ending the day feeling energised.
Feeling happy most of the time.
Feeling confident most of the time.

GOOD HEALTH . . .

makes you happier
gives you more energy
reduces your disease risk
increases your lifespan.

THE INSIDE STORY

What is *your* idea of good health?

....

....

....

....

....

....

....

....

....

....

....

....

....

....

....

#4
WHAT INFLUENCES YOUR HEALTH?

Health doesn't stay the same all through your life. It changes through time, and it's influenced by a lot of different factors, including genes, work, money, organisation, friends and family, and knowledge. All of these things can influence your health for better or worse, depending on how you act.

YOUR GENES

Your genes determine a lot about your life, but they don't rule with an iron fist. We all have the ability to work within the limits imposed by our genes - we just need to know what to do and how to do it. Our genes provide the script, but we've got the ability to improvise!

YOUR WORK

For most of us, work occupies a lot of our time and because of that it can have a huge influence on our health. If you're in a job where you sit in front of a computer screen all day, then you're going to be burning much less energy than someone who builds houses. However, this doesn't mean you should think everything's hopeless so you might as well give up! Instead, look for things that you *can* control. Can you park the car further away from the office, so that you get to walk a bit more? Could you cycle to work? Can you alternate standing and sitting at work? Can you organise walking meetings instead of sitting down together in an airless room? Can you volunteer for tasks that you know will allow you to move more?

In most cases it's possible to figure out ways to change up your work environment – even if they're minor changes – to help you live more healthily.

YOUR MONEY

You don't need a lot of money to be healthy. For sure, having money makes it easier to buy healthy food – but it also makes it easier to buy unhealthy food! Having money means that you can splash out on a ritzy gym membership (and then feel guilty about not going) – but you don't need that gym to get exercise. Some of the unhealthiest people around are those who have big incomes: they spend so much time working and chasing money that they forget to look after the one thing that's more valuable than cash – their health.

HOW ORGANISED YOU ARE

Even more than genes, work and money put together, a lack of organisation will seriously affect your health. If you're not organised, how will you find the time to exercise? How will you be able to shop for good food? How will you be able to prepare healthy meals and snacks? If you spend most of your life lurching crazily from one crisis to the next, your health is going to suffer.

Not everyone is a naturally super-organised supremo, but we can all add a bit more planning and structure into our day. And as we become more organised, we free up more time to do the things we want – including looking after our health.

YOUR FRIENDS AND FAMILY

Good friends and good family are great to have in your life – but sometimes they can really mess up your efforts to be healthy. Who hasn't gone out for a meal with friends and eaten twice as much as they would normally? How often do you catch up with a friend for coffee and, between you, decide that cake's a great idea too? Or get together for a family meal and graze on endless bags of potato chips and peanuts while the dinner's cooking?

SIZE + SCALE

WE ALL LOVE FOOD. THAT'S WIRED INTO
OUR GENES. IF I DIDN'T FOCUS ON MY
HEALTH AND HOW I EAT, THEN I COULD
EASILY WEIGH 120 KG. I WILL NEVER WEIGH
70 KG – AT LEAST, NOT A HEALTHY 70 KG.
BUT IT *IS* REALISTIC FOR ME TO WEIGH IN
AT 90 KG, AS LONG AS I PAY ATTENTION
TO HOW I LIVE. MY GENES PUT ME AT THE
HEAVIER END OF THE SCALE FOR A NEW
ZEALAND MALE – BUT *I* GET TO SAY JUST
HOW FAR ALONG THAT SCALE I SIT.

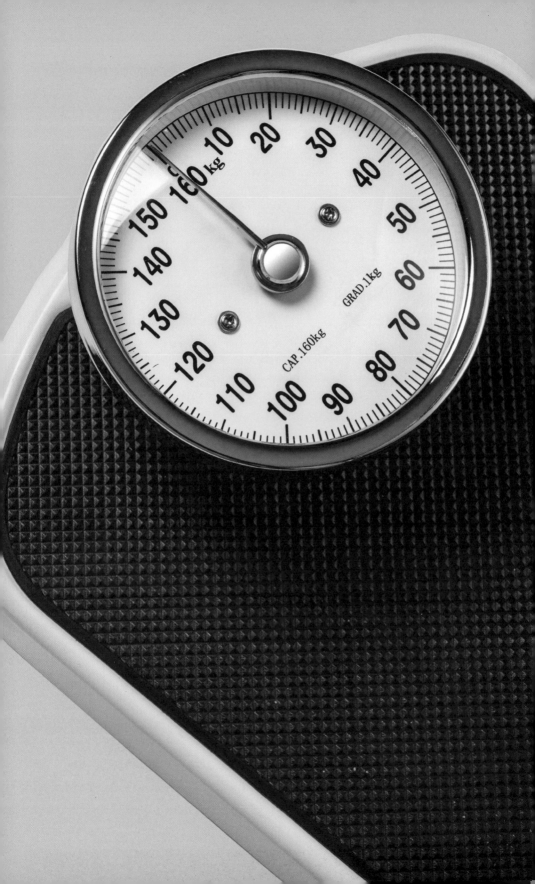

Food is such a strong expression of love that it's hard to say no when someone who cares about you has prepared a delicious, tasty meal. It occurs in all cultures, and even more so in Maori and Pacific Island families. This wouldn't be a problem if food was scarce, but that's not the world we live in today. Most of us have access to too much food too much of the time. Those feasts can happen far too often, with terrible consequences for your health.

YOUR KNOWLEDGE

Probably the biggest *single* influence on your health is how much knowledge you have about food itself. If you don't know what foods do to your body, how can you possibly make good choices?

To make things harder, there are thousands of people out there who will tell you what to do – but most of them contradict each other, which just leaves you totally confused. Do you eat a high-fat diet – or a low-fat one? Do you focus on wholegrain foods, or do you leave them out altogether? Maybe you should go Paleo, and mainly eat meat? Or perhaps you should be vegan and shun all animal products? Ah, maybe you should be vegan after 6 pm; then again, maybe you should fast two days a week and eat what you want the rest of the time. And look, these people are selling a magic pill that will stop you craving food and help you lose 10 kg in 10 days . . .

And it's not just food advice that's confusing – just take a look at the different messages around exercise. You can choose from low-intensity cardio (like walking) or high-intensity cardio (like running) – or you could do high-intensity interval training (HIIT). Or maybe you need to do resistance work, and get the weights out. Maybe yoga is the answer. Or Pilates? Or yogalates?

All of these different approaches to food and fitness can easily be found on the internet, in magazines and in books. And each one of them will be right for someone. But which one is right for *you*? If you have enough knowledge to assess the different approaches and see which one works for you, then you'll be well on the way to developing your own personal plan for a healthy, positive life.

#5 HOW THIS BOOK CAN HELP

Many health and fitness books will give you a prescription – eat this food, do this exercise, and you'll be happy and healthy, just like the author. And sometimes, that works. But the fact that many of us are still getting fatter and sicker is a pretty clear sign that it's not working for everyone.

The problem with a prescription is that it doesn't take into account the unique challenges of *your* life. It doesn't deal with *your* likes or dislikes, *your* financial situation, what sort of work *you* do, how much time *you* have available, or what social and family obligations *you* have. If it doesn't fit into *your* life, then it's not likely to be much use to you in the long run.

This book won't give you a prescription. Instead, it will give you the *knowledge* that you need to build your own personal health and fitness plan – one that works with the life that you lead.

   # You'll consider why you want to change – you'll find out which aspects of good health are important to you.

   # You'll learn how your body works, so that you can understand the effect that good and poor health has on it.

   # You'll learn about nutrition basics, and about how to build a way of eating and fuelling your body that works for you.

   # You'll learn about a range of tactics that you can use to apply all of this information to your life, so that you build new, healthy habits that you can sustain.

   # And, last of all, you'll get to put it all together into your own personal action plan – something that you can use to get the healthy lifestyle you're looking for.

So dive in, and find out how to become your own health guru.

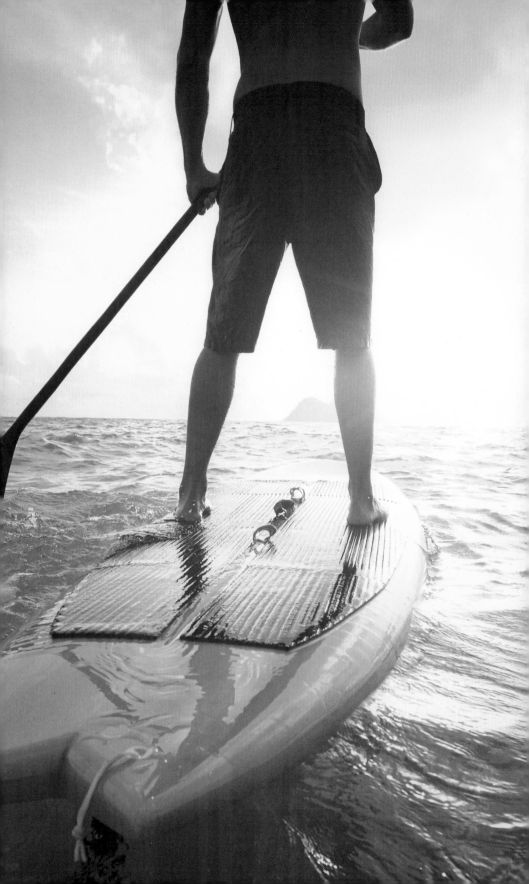

PART TWO
—
INSIDE YOUR HEART

In today's hyper-connected world, it can feel like there's always someone telling us how we should feel. Every social media platform has an 'inspo' element to it — from clean eating bowls of exotic (and expensive) ingredients, to perfectly presented physiques on pristine beaches, to adrenaline-fuelled adventure addicts posting from some obscure part of the planet. Even if you know that what you're seeing is not the truth, the whole truth and nothing but the truth, it's still a bit demoralising. In reality — it doesn't matter. It's someone else's life. What does matter is your life and your goals. To figure out what these are, you need to stop looking to the outside world, and start looking inwards.

#6 WHY DO YOU WANT TO CHANGE?

When it comes to looking after our health, we all tend to fall into one of two categories. Either we're very aware of how we're doing, checking in with ourselves regularly to see if we need to change anything; or we're just trucking on with life, not paying any attention to our health until something dramatic happens. You'll know which camp you fall into.

If you're in the 'she'll be right' group – and have recently discovered that she might just be wrong – then you're probably not used to deliberately making changes to improve your health. And you're probably thinking that this is going to be hard. The one thing that's really going to help you here is knowing exactly *why* you want to change.

You're unlikely to change because your doctor said you should, or because you watched a TV programme about the effects of obesity, or because you read something about the soaring rates of diabetes worldwide. These things are important, sure, but they're not things that normally motivate us to change our lives. What we all need is a *personal* reason to change – something that we can hang on to when the going gets tough. We're all going to have our own reasons for wanting to be healthy, but here are a few that crop up fairly regularly. Take a look at them to see which ones apply to you.

REASONS FOR WANTING TO BE HEALTHY

   # I want to have more energy every day.
   # I want to be healthy enough to play with my grandkids.
   # I need to be able to pass my medical for work.
   # I want to be able to live my life without limitations.

I've got a family history of heart disease/cancer/diabetes

\#   I've got a family history of heart disease/cancer/diabetes and I want to minimise my chances of going through that.

\#   I want to be able to run a marathon/climb a mountain/ complete a 100 km cycle race.

\#   I don't want to feel so tired every morning.

\#   I want to lose weight.

\#   I want to look hot and be an Instagram star.

\#   I think my health is stopping me earning good money.

\#   I don't want to end up frail and weak when I'm older.

\#   I want to be a role model for my kids.

YOUR REASONS FOR WANTING TO CHANGE

When you're thinking about *your* motivation to change your health, ask yourself this: 'Who cares?'

Do you? If not, does your family? Would your children, partner, brothers, sisters, parents be upset if you ended up suffering from a preventable illness or disorder that was triggered by your unhealthy lifestyle? Do your friends care? Does your employer?

Sometimes, having another person in your health equation really helps – especially when it's a rainy day and you have to get out of bed and go for a run, or when you're facing the third morning-tea shout of the week at work!

Take some time to really think about why you want to change and what – or who – is going to motivate you. Write it down somewhere. It doesn't matter where you write it – on a huge sheet of paper stuck on the fridge, on a tiny note stuck to the corner of your bathroom mirror, or as a secret sentence somewhere on your phone. It can be clear or cryptic, words or pictures, short or long – all that matters is that it works for you and that you can see it when you need it.

Why do you need to change?

....

....

#7 WHAT DO YOU WANT TO CHANGE?

This is pretty basic: if you want to achieve something, you *have* to know what it is! We're all great at saying 'I'd love to be fitter', 'I wish I weighed less', 'I want to be stronger'. But we can never achieve those goals, because they totally lack an endpoint.

Goals with a clear destination are harder to come up with, but easier to achieve. It's much easier to say 'I want to be fitter' than 'I want to be fit enough to run a 10 km race in March'. That second statement commits you to a goal – even if you only say it to yourself.

You might have several goals, in which case clarifying them and writing them down is even more important. Applying timeframes can help, too. If you're not sure what your goals are, here are some examples to consider.

SOME MEASURABLE GOALS

- # I want to reduce my waist circumference by 2 cm.
- # I want my waist circumference to be less than half my height.
- # I want to do 20 minutes of exercise every day.
- # I want to stop taking sugar in my tea/coffee/hot chocolate.
- # I want to eat a high-protein, high-fat, low-carb breakfast five days out of seven.
- # I want to only eat in a 12-hour window.
- # I want to be strong enough to do 20 full-body push-ups.
- # I want to be able to run a 5 km race in less than 30 minutes.

MAKING YOUR GOALS REALISTIC

Once you've identified your goal or goals, stop for a moment and think about how you got to where you are right now. If you're carrying more weight than you'd like, think about when you were last happy with how much you weighed. How long did it take for you to get from there to where you are now? It's important to know how long that journey was, because the return journey is likely to be just as long.

  # If you've put on 20 kg over the past two years, you're not going to lose that in two months.

  # If you get out of breath going up a single flight of stairs, you're not going to be able to run a 5 km race two weeks from now.

Knowing that this is a lifestyle change, not a temporary sticking plaster, is important when deciding what you want to change.

What are your goals?

....

....

....

....

....

....

....

....

#8 WHAT'S STOPPING YOU CHANGING?

We're all creatures of habit – and that can be a good thing or a bad thing, depending on the habit! Changing habits is challenging, but not impossible. We do it often enough when we have to, but less often when there isn't an immediate, compelling need. For instance, if you learnt to drive in a manual car but later on buy an automatic, you have to change your habit of using a gearstick. It takes a few goes, but you get it pretty quickly. We also make bigger changes: if you start a family, for example, you're very likely to stop partying all weekend, staying up late every night, or spending all your spare cash on fun little things.

Situations like these involve an extrinsic motivating factor – a trigger that's outside of us, separate from us. The gearstick in the car just isn't there for us to use any more, so we have to change; the new baby is part of our lives all of a sudden, so again we have to change. An extrinsic trigger makes it a bit easier for us to change, because, really, we're forced into it. We don't have much choice. We might not always like the changes we have to make, but we can achieve them most of the time.

The difference with choosing to live a healthy lifestyle is that it *is* a choice. We don't *have* to do it. We can continue to eat what we like, drink what we like, slob around on the sofa and binge-watch TV all weekend, every weekend, if that's what we want. We're all adults; there's nobody telling us what to do. So, if we're going to choose a healthy lifestyle, we need *intrinsic* motivation to help us succeed. That's really what we were looking at in the section '*What* do you want to change?' (see page 29).

When it comes to changing your lifestyle and choosing to live more healthily, having a strong intrinsic motivation is critical to your success. You need to bring this motivation into the picture when your life puts up barriers to change – and this will happen a lot!

Each of us has different things in our life that make it difficult for us to stick to a healthy lifestyle. It might be habits that we learnt from our parents; our financial situation; time pressures; the people we live or socialise with; or a voice inside our head that constantly tells us to take the easy option. All of these are potential barriers to change – but as long as you're aware of them, you can overcome them. Below are some examples of common roadblocks, and ways that they can be addressed.

PEOPLE WHO ENCOURAGE YOUR BAD HABITS

These are often friends you love spending time with. They're the ones who'll say things like 'Come on, let's get another bottle of wine', or 'Right, we've walked for 20 minutes – we've earned an ice cream'. You might have become friends in the first place because of your common love of indulgent food or good wine, so it's natural for you to do these things when you're together. And it's OK if this is a 'sometimes' activity. The problem starts when it's a regular thing and is interfering with your efforts to be healthier.

Solution: You don't want to ruin your friendship, so what do you do? One option is to suggest an alternative – rather than going for more wine, you might say you'd prefer a coffee right now. Your friend can, of course, still have the wine. True friends are not likely to be offended and you'll still have a great time together.

The other place bad habits get encouraged is in the home. Your significant other – your partner, your husband, your wife – loves you and likes to express that by buying things you enjoy. This might be chocolate, wine or Friday-night fish and chips – any treat you find hard to resist.

Solution: Good communication skills can help here! You don't want to upset your loved one – after all, they've just done something nice for you. At the same time, however, you want to discourage them from doing this quite so often. How you go about this will probably depend on your relationship and the way you naturally communicate with each other, but as a general rule it's probably worth thanking them for being so thoughtful and then, later, gently suggesting a healthier alternative.

PEOPLE WHO SHOW LOVE BY FEEDING YOU

This is usually done by family, and it's most likely going to be your mother. Providing food for family members is a fundamental human behaviour, and it's just so easy for parents to take the 'some is good so more is better' approach. You're much more at risk of this derailing your health efforts if you live near your family and you get together frequently. Whether it's lunch or dinner, the table will be stacked with food, and plates will be piled high – with second helpings being almost compulsory.

Solution: The good thing here is that your family is probably going to love you no matter what, so you can sit down and have a chat with them to explain why you're not keen on having so much food. You could say something like 'Look, Mum, I know you love me and that's why you make all this delicious food, because you want me to be happy. But if I eat too much I'm not going to be as healthy as I want. And I really want to be healthy so that I can be around for a long time – I bet you want that too. So if I don't eat as much as you think I should, it's not because I don't like your cooking – it's because I want to have a long, healthy life so that I can be around to look after you when you're older.'

WORK ISSUES

'I'm too busy with work' is probably the most widely used excuse when it comes to changing our health habits. And for most people, it really *is* just an excuse. Yes, you might be spending 2 hours a day commuting and 8 hours a day working or studying, but that still leaves 14 hours. Sleep for 8 of those and you still have 6 left over. What you do with those 6 hours can make a huge difference to your health.

Solutions: During your 6 hours of free time, you could prepare healthy meals to take to work – for both breakfast and lunch, if necessary. You could do some exercise (by yourself, or with family or friends), instead of just sitting on the couch watching TV. You could do some chores, so that on the weekend you'd be free to go and enjoy yourself doing fun activities.

It might also be possible to build some exercise in to your commute. Could you get off the bus a few stops earlier or park the car further away from your premises, and so get in a bit of walking? At lunchtime, do you have to sit at your desk or could you get outside for a walk? If you're in an office, do you have to send emails to your colleagues or could you get up and walk over to see them?

In many workplaces the biggest threat to a healthy lifestyle is those endless morning teas where kind-hearted colleagues bring in cakes and savouries to share. There are several ways to deal with these.

Solutions: You can try bringing in a healthy option, such as hummus or salsa with carrot and celery sticks for dipping. If someone else has provided the food, you can just take a small piece and nibble on it slowly so that it lasts for the length of the morning tea. Another strategy is to pat your stomach and say 'I had a massive breakfast this morning and I'm still full. It looks delicious, but I just couldn't manage anything right now.'

MONEY ISSUES

Having less disposable income than some others can make it seem impossible to live a healthy lifestyle with plenty of exercise. It's not – but it takes a bit more thought, and maybe a bit more time, than if you have spare cash to spend. It's worth keeping in mind that you don't *need* to join a gym or buy expensive workout clothes to get to a level of physical fitness that will benefit your health.

Solutions: Going for a walk is a perfectly good aerobic activity – as long as you walk fast enough to get your heart rate up a bit. No dawdling so that you take 30 minutes to walk a kilometre! You can also do strength training and flexibility exercises at home, with very little or no equipment. Your bodyweight is often all you need to provide enough resistance to help you build muscle strength. There are heaps of exercise examples in the 'Functional Fitness for All' section on page 52.

Choosing healthy food is also often seen as impossible if you don't have a lot of money. It's really common to read that takeaways, bread and potatoes are the only options for people on a tight budget. Many news and lifestyle websites quote studies showing that healthy food is far more expensive than unhealthy options. However, some of these studies look at the price per 100 g of a particular food, while others look at the price per calorie. Only a few look at the price *per serving* of healthy options versus their less healthy equivalents – like a wholegrain sourdough loaf versus the cheapest supermarket white sliced bread. That means these studies don't really translate to the real world so easily.

Solutions: In fact, low-cost cooking is currently being touted as one of the healthiest ways to eat. *Cucina povera*, which translates as 'food of the poor', is traditional Italian fare. It uses fresh vegetables, herbs, olive oil, legumes, fish and a little bit of meat, along with pasta and bread. As money was scarce in the communities where *cucina povera* originated, the food was seasonal – because when something is in season, it's at its cheapest, and often at its best too! If you want to keep your food costs down and your nutritional value up, you can follow similar principles. Eat seasonally, and eat close to the beginning of the food chain.

ENERGY-SUCKERS

Warning! You or someone you know could be sucking the energy out of your life – and it will be your health that suffers. Ever find yourself going 'I *caaan't* . . .', in the sort of sad, whiny tone that three-year-olds specialise in? Or 'It hurts', 'It's too hard', 'I don't want to'. There are dozens of riffs on this theme, but underneath they're all the same. Energy-sucking excuses that we use to stop us tackling things that really matter, but that take effort to achieve.

Then there are the other people who suck the energy out of us. We've all met people who view life as a pit of misery and despair. They trudge through the day, dragging their load of negativity around with them, knocking the joy out of other people's lives. The only thing they have energy for is telling you – and anyone else – how tough their life is, how much everything hurts, and why they can't possibly do anything about it. Being exposed to such a negative attitude day in, day out takes its toll on us. It's hard not to be affected by all this negativity, especially when you're trying to make changes to your own behaviour.

Solution: If you're your own energy-sucker, the only way to tackle this is probably to take a long, hard look in the mirror and tell yourself that you deserve better.

Solution: Spending too much time in the company of energy-sapping individuals will bring you down and harm your chances of developing a healthier, stronger you. The only thing you can do is to avoid contact as often as possible. If an energy-sucker starts dumping on you, give them a bright, chipper 'Gosh, that's terrible for you' and excuse yourself right away: 'Sorry, I've got to go and pick up the kids/go to a meeting/get to my yoga class.' Offering them solutions – 'Have you tried Pilates?' – will only elicit a dozen more reasons why they can't do that. Ultimately, their attitude and their health is *their* responsibility, not yours. Save your energy for looking after yourself.

THE VOICE INSIDE YOUR HEAD

If there's one thing that's going to stop you changing, it's the voice inside your head. You know the one – it says things like this:

\# 'That big pack of biscuits (or chocolate, potato chips, etc.) is better value – you should get that one.'

 # 'It's too cold/wet/windy – give your walk/run/bike ride a miss today.'
 # 'Stay in bed this morning – don't get up and do your exercises.'
 # 'It's too much effort to cook – get takeaways instead.'
 # 'Yeah it's late, but just watch one more episode of *Game of Thrones* before you go to bed.'
 # 'You're not paying for this food, so you may as well eat as much as you can.'

This is the voice that helped you become less healthy than you wanted. Unless you learn how to shut it down, it's going to take you even further down the same path. None of us is ever going to get rid of that voice – it's part of us – but we *can* learn to recognise it and stop it dominating our lives.

What does your voice say to you?

....

....

....

....

....

....

....

....

....

SILENCING THE VOICE INSIDE YOUR HEAD

The first step is to acknowledge that it's there. It is perfectly normal to have an inner dialogue going on. We debate with ourselves all the time – 'Shall I leave for work now, or spend another 10 minutes on Twitter?' 'Do I have to mow the lawn today, or can I leave it till next week?' 'Hmm, meal deal or just the burger?' The voice in your head presents you with options, all the time.

Next, identify situations where you know that the voice inside your head will try to convince you to do something that's not in line with your health goals. It might be in relation to food, to exercise, to sleep, or to something else. Take some time to really visualise this:

See yourself in the supermarket, standing in the confectionary aisle. You're looking at the chocolate bars and hearing that voice encouraging you to buy one (or two, 'cos they're on special, you know?).

See yourself getting home from work and pouring a glass of wine before dinner, then hearing that voice telling you to get another to go with your meal – and another one later on, because you've had a hard day, after all.

See yourself waking up in the morning, reaching for your phone and spending an hour on social media – while the voice in your head says, 'It'll be fine, you can exercise tonight.'

The more realistic you can make these images, the better, because then you're more likely to be aware of these situations when they occur in real life. Creating awareness is a big part of actually overcoming that voice inside your head.

Now, think about how you could respond in each of those situations. If you find yourself in the chocolate aisle, can you tell yourself 'I don't want this today' and then just walk away? If you get home and pour a glass of wine, can you say 'I'll just wait and have that with dinner', and then drink it slowly so that it lasts longer? When you wake up in the morning, can you limit yourself to 15 minutes on social media, and then get up and exercise?

As our reactions are usually automatic, it can help to have a 'time out' period between hearing the voice and doing what it tells you. Think of this like a set of traffic lights: red is 'Uh-oh, the voice is talking'; amber is 'I'm going to slow down and assess the situation'; green is 'I'm going to take this action.' Some ideas for 'amber-light activities' are:

Count to 10 – slowly!
Take three breaths, focusing on the feeling of the air moving in and out of your body.
Recite your 'Why I want to change' mantra (see page 28).
Think about those who care whether you change or not.
Visualise the consequences of your decision – will it make you more healthy, or less?

Hitting the pause button on your actions will help you make better choices. It won't happen straight away, but after a while it will take less effort to make the choice that supports your long-term goals, rather than the one that meets your short-term desires.

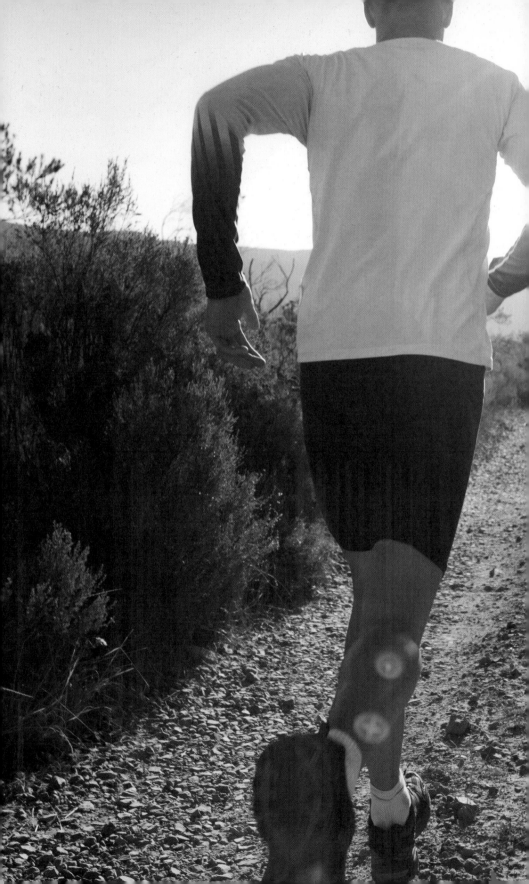

PART THREE

—

UNDER YOUR SKIN

The first step towards getting healthy is understanding how your body is built, how the food you eat and the way you move — or don't move — affect it.

The old saying 'you are what you eat' is so true. If you eat junk all the time, you're simply not going to build a strong, healthy body. You need to put the right stuff in to get a body that will hold up against everything you throw at it. It's like building a house: try doing that with some driftwood, some pine cones and a bit of moss — you're really not going to get a good result. Build with concrete and bricks and treated timber, instead, and you'll get something that will stand the test of time.

#9 THEM BONES

WHAT YOUR BODY DOES

Although they're hidden from view, our bones still sometimes get the blame for excess weight. You've probably heard a few people say 'I'm just big-boned.' And it's true that bone size does vary – the size, shape and strength of your bones are in part determined by your genes. If both of your parents are tall, chances are you will be, too. If both of your parents are short, then you're more likely to be below average height. But lifestyle and environment also help to shape our bones. An example of this is that good nutrition when you're young will probably mean you'll end up taller than your parents.

Our bones are living tissue – that's why they can heal if we break them. Even when our bones aren't broken, our bodies remove old, damaged bone tissue and replace it with new, stronger bone. This is called bone remodelling. It helps to ensure that your skeleton can support your weight and resist moderate shocks from falls and minor accidents.

Like all living tissue, bones change over time. When you're very young, your bones are quite flexible. As you get older, they become stiffer, stronger and more resilient. But then, as you move towards old age, your bones can become weaker and more fragile, particularly as a result of osteoporosis. This develops when minerals such as calcium are lost from your bones faster than your body can replace them. Osteoporosis increases the risk of fractures. It's a problem for both women and men, and the risk starts to increase once you're over 50.

DID YOU KNOW?

Most of the adult skeleton is replaced every 10 years.

FIT:5

Food for your bones

1. Focus on lean proteins, good fats, colourful fruit and veges.
2. Include good sources of calcium, like dairy and tinned fish (with the bones).
3. Eat a variety of foods – don't restrict your diet or focus on one type of food.
4. Keep it unprocessed – you'll get far more of the nutrients you need and much less of the salt you don't need.
5. Get regular exposure to the sun – without risking sunburn. Sunscreen will stop vitamin D being made, so make sure to get some of your sun exposure when the UV index is low enough to go outside without protection.

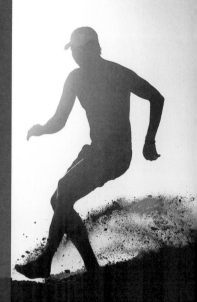

DID YOU KNOW?

Rickets is a bone disorder caused by poor diet and lack of vitamin D. As long ago as the early 1700s, cod liver oil and exposure to sun were used to treat the disease. It's recently started to appear again in the UK!

WHAT YOU CAN DO

If you want to have strong bones – regardless of your age – then you should think about what you eat and how you exercise.

FEED YOUR BONES

The two bone-health nutrients that get the most attention are calcium and vitamin D.

Calcium gets a lot of attention because studies – mainly in the US – have shown that most people don't get enough calcium in their diet. The dieting fads of the past few decades meant that people were avoiding dairy-based foods because of their fat content – but as a result they were losing out on some important nutrients, including calcium.

Vitamin D helps the body absorb calcium. We get vitamin D in particular foods, but it's also made by our bodies when we are out in the sunlight. As we've become more aware of the dangers of too much sun – or maybe as we just spend more time in front of screens – fewer of us are getting enough vitamin D.

It's not just these two things that keep our bones healthy:

Phosphorus and magnesium are essential for forming hydroxyapatite, the main building block of our bones.

Vitamin C, vitamin K, copper, manganese, zinc and iron all play a part in the processes that build our bones.

45

\# Having enough potassium in your diet helps to reduce calcium loss from your bones; having too much sodium increases calcium loss – another reason not to go overboard with the salt!

If you tried to regulate all this using supplements and multi-vitamins, you'd get into all sorts of difficulties. The best way to look after bone health is to eat a healthy diet, with lean protein, good fats, and colourful fruit and vegetables. *If you look after your diet, your body will look after your bones.*

STRENGTHEN YOUR BONES

The other thing you need for strong bones is a bit of regular stress. Not the sort of stress that makes you want to reach for a glass of wine, but the physical stress that comes from exercise.

Your body is constantly monitoring how much stress is being placed on your bones. When you do things that require your body to resist forces – so, any activity that involves impact – your body reacts to this by increasing the strength of your bones. Specialised cells called osteoclasts remove tiny areas of bone that have damage, like little cracks. Then another type of cell – an osteoblast – comes in and puts in new bone material so that the bone is stronger. If this didn't happen, over time you'd end up with weak, brittle bones.

While putting stress on your bones encourages your body to perform this remodelling, it's something that has to be done regularly to be effective. You can't expect to get strong bones by going for a walk once a month – your body needs to get the 'strengthen me' message every couple of days.

DID YOU KNOW?

The reason why men are generally taller than women is because oestrogen inhibits bone lengthening – and women have a lot more oestrogen than men.

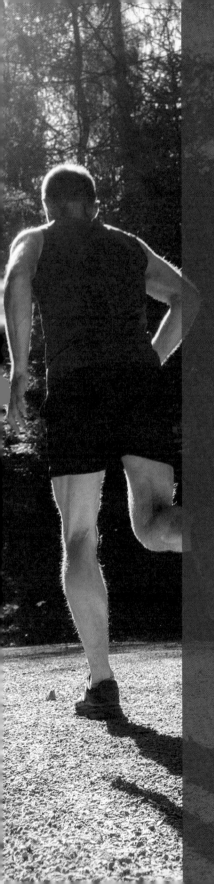

FIT:5

Bone-friendly exercises

1. Walking – if you do this outside, you'll also get vitamin D
2. Jogging or running
3. Skipping
4. Dancing
5. Weight-lifting or resistance exercises for the upper body

#10 THE SOFT- TISSUE STORY

WHAT YOUR BODY DOES

Just as your bones are influenced by your genetics and the lifestyle you lead (see previous section 'Them Bones'), so are your muscles. Your gender has the biggest effect on how big your muscles can get – as a rule, women generally have smaller, less bulky muscles than men. This is because testosterone drives muscle formation – and men have far more testosterone than women. A 30-year-old man will typically have a testosterone level of 270–1070 ng/dL, while a woman of the same age will have only 15–70 ng/dL. In other words, a woman has only about 6% of the testosterone of a man – so she has virtually no chance of ever looking like Arnie or The Rock.

Testosterone also affects muscle strength, but so does physical activity. An office worker who doesn't do any physical work won't be as strong as their colleague who cycles to work, goes to the gym three days a week and spends a lot of time working in the garden on the weekends. This is because your muscles respond to physical stress, just like your bones do. The way they respond depends on the type of stress you put on them.

\# At the gym, if you're lifting weights that are just a bit heavier than you can comfortably manage, you'll be stressing the neuromuscular system. Your body detects this stress. One response is to activate cells called satellite cells. These are a type of stem cell, which means that they can turn into other cells when they get the right signal. When they get the go-ahead from your body, the satellite cells start multiplying. Some of them turn into myoblasts, which fuse with existing muscle tissue and both repair it and increase the size of the muscle. In non-scientific language, basically your body thinks: 'Hmm, these weights are heavy, I need to make bigger, stronger muscles to cope with them', and then sets about doing just that.

\# Say that, instead, you run very long distances, day after day after day. Now your body doesn't want large muscles – because this means a lot of extra weight to carry around, and your body wants to expend as little energy as necessary while it's doing all this running. It does, however, want the ability to produce lots of energy in your muscles. It does this by increasing the number of mitochondria in your muscle cells. Mitochondria are like little power units: they burn glucose and fatty acids that are produced from our food, and so supply the energy that makes your muscles contract (along with fuelling a whole host of other metabolic processes). And it's not just running – any type of endurance exercise will produce this effect.

Now, these aren't one-way systems. If you lift weights for a week and then never touch them again, you're not going to keep any muscle growth that you achieved. If you train to run one marathon in your twenties and then spend the next 10 years sitting on the couch, all of those extra mitochondria you had are going to die off. When it comes to muscle strength and mitochondria, if you don't use it, then you're going to lose it.

WHAT YOU CAN DO

When it comes to being healthy, most of us are after a balance. We want muscles that are strong but can also go the distance, so that we can run or walk or swim as long as we like. To get this, we need to do a variety of exercise, and do it consistently. If we only do one exercise, then yes, we'll get good at it – but overall we won't be balanced. If you just focus on lifting weights then you'll easily be able to pick up your kids – but you might not be able to catch them!

BUILD EXERCISE INTO YOUR DAY

Fortunately, a lot of exercise can actually be built into your day – you don't have to 'do' exercise in a certain way for a certain amount of time. Little and often is a great way to get your daily exercise. Check out the 'Fit 5' opposite for some ideas on how to integrate more activity into your day. What else would work for you?

DO FUNCTIONAL EXERCISE

It's also important to know that your body doesn't work like a series of isolated muscle movements. Your body is much more fluid – your muscles work in a coordinated way that produces actual functional movements like standing up, walking around, and bending down to pick something up. Think about the simple act of moving from the couch to the kitchen to get a cup of tea and a biscuit, then sitting down again to watch TV. There are dozens of movements involved – and none of them look anything like a bicep curl.

These functional movement patterns, which we use every day, developed as we evolved as a species. They're hard-wired into our brains. The problem is that we don't use them anywhere near as much now as we did even 50 years ago. We sit in a car to go to work, we sit at a desk all day, we sit in a café to eat our lunch, we sit in a car to come home, and we sit on a sofa to eat our dinner and watch TV. And guess what happens? Our bodies forget how to move. Our glutes switch off, our core becomes weak, our back muscles atrophy. We hunch and slump our way through the day, setting ourselves up for a future that's likely to include disability and distress.

Luckily, you can do something about this. Including an exercise programme that's built on functional movements that will re-educate your body and help return it to a strong, healthy state. You can build a body that will serve you well today and will also set you up for a healthy, active life in future years. To see how you can do this, take a look at the 'Functional Fitness for All' section on page 52.

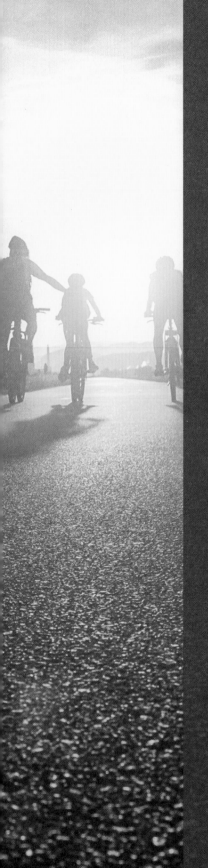

FIT:5

Built-in exercise

1. At work, the mall or the supermarket, park your car well away from the entrance and benefit from the extra bit of walking. Once you're inside, take the stairs, not the elevator or escalator.
2. Stand, don't sit. Whenever possible, stand up when you're talking on the phone, talking to people, even when you're eating a meal.
3. Wash your car yourself, rather than taking it through the carwash at the petrol station – you'll get an all-over upper-body workout.
4. Housework is actually great full-body exercise – even better if you put on some music and dance around as you do it!
5. If you've got a garden, get out into it. If you're paying someone else to look after it, *they're* getting the exercise, not you.

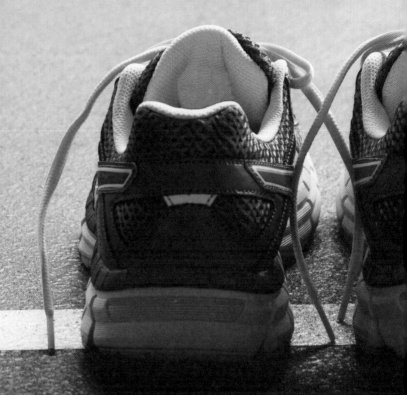

FUNCTIONAL FITNESS FOR ALL

BUILD STRENGTH

The table opposite shows you a go-to exercise routine for building a strong, lean and healthy body in a short time, without needing to spend all day at the gym! It consists of five functional movement patterns: push (pressing away from you), pull (tugging towards you), hip-hinge (bending from the middle), squat (flexing at the knee and hip) and pillar (stabilising your core). You simply pick one exercise from each section, do 10-12 reps of each, and repeat until you have completed three sets.

This is an incredibly efficient routine – it will give your muscles a great workout, and help you get more strength and a faster metabolism quickly. You don't need a gym, either – each category has bodyweight exercises you can do at home. As you get stronger, you can add some simple home-based equipment, or you can go all out and join a gym – the options are there for you.

To see descriptions of all of the exercises, turn to page 244 (Functional Fitness for All – Extras).

FUNCTIONAL PICK-'N'-MIX

If you want to keep track of which functional exercises you are doing, make a copy of this table and tick off the ones you're currently focusing on. Exercises marked with a * require gym equipment.

PUSH			
Static lunge		Classic push-up	
Forward lunge		Kneeling push-up	
Reverse lunge		Elevated push-up	
Walking lunge		Hand-release push-up	
Side lunge		Pike push-up	
Bulgarian split squat		Wall push-up	
Bench press*		Single-leg push-up	
Standard shoulder press*			
Arnie shoulder press*			
PULL			
TYIW		Dumbbell row*	
Pull-up		Suspension trainer row*	
Horizontal pull-up		Lat pulldown*	
		Seated row*	
HIP-HINGE			
Good morning		Deadlift with barbell*	
Single leg Romanian deadlift		Kettlebell swing*	
Hip thrust		Romanian deadlift with barbell*	
Frog squat		Barbell hip thrust*	
SQUAT			
Squat			
PILLAR			
High plank		Crunch	
Low plank		Reverse crunch	
Side plank			

FIT:5

Home help

You don't really *need* equipment to do exercise, but it can help if you want to mix things up. So if you're looking to build a home gym, start with these five items:

1. Your body - no matter how fit you are, bodyweight exercises will make you even fitter.
2. A circuit timer - go high-tech and download a free app for your phone, or just use a cheap kitchen timer.
3. A suspension trainer - these consist of a number of straps or ropes that anchor to a strong point (like a door or a tree). A good suspension trainer lets you use your bodyweight in a wide range of exercises.
4. A heavy resistance band - good for working on larger muscles, like your legs and glutes.
5. A light resistance band - good for working on smaller muscles, like your arms and shoulders.

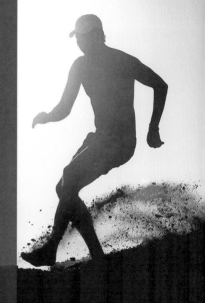

#11 BEAT BOX

WHAT YOUR BODY DOES

Think about your heart. It's been beating since before you were born, and it will continue to do so until the day you die. Your heart is made of muscle – but it's not the same as the muscle that makes up your impressive abs or your toned legs.

Your heart is made of a special type of muscle called cardiac muscle. The fibres making up this muscle are highly connected with each other, which helps them to react together in a wave of activity – this is what causes the beating motion of your heart. The rate at which your heart beats is controlled by specialised cells called pacemaker cells. When you get anxious, or when you run or get stressed or get scared, these cells tell the heart to beat faster. This sends more oxygenated blood shooting round your body, which helps your body get ready to respond to whatever threat you're facing.

How hard your heart has to work depends on a number of factors.

Weight plays a big part – the more excess weight you carry, the further the blood has to travel around your body, so the harder the heart has to work.

The elasticity of your blood vessels also affects the heart's workload – stiffer blood vessels are less efficient at moving blood through the body, so the heart has to pump harder. Stiffer blood vessels cause an increase in blood pressure.

Your heart is also affected by the quality of its oxygen supply. It's a muscle, and it needs a steady supply of oxygen to work. This oxygen gets supplied by blood that flows through your coronary arteries. When one or more of these gets blocked, oxygen supply to the heart is reduced and the cells die. This is known as a myocardial infarction – or a heart attack, in common language.

Since the heart is a muscle, it will become stronger with exercise. If you have had an active lifestyle for many years, the muscle fibres in your heart will be bigger. Each beat of your heart is therefore stronger, so fewer beats are required at rest – and your heart is better able to cope with a sudden need for speed, too. Regular exercise helps your body make more branches and connections between the coronary arteries, so if one artery becomes constricted then blood can still get to the tissues via other routes.

WHAT YOU CAN DO

Since you need your heart to stay alive, it makes a lot of sense to look after it! Fortunately, it's not that difficult if you're interested in having a healthy lifestyle.

YOU CAN EXERCISE

Physical exercise will definitely help keep your ticker in good nick. The good news is that you don't have to go out and run an ultramarathon, or do an Ironman or row across the Pacific Ocean. To benefit your heart, you only have to do moderate exercise. This means a level that allows you to have enough puff left to talk, but not enough to sing.

Walking is good. Brisk walking is great – but it *must* be brisk. A slow dawdle round the shops doesn't count as heart-healthy exercise – especially if your destination is the food court! A jog is fantastic. Cycling is also good, as is swimming, running, rowing, kayaking or any other aerobic exercise that you enjoy and can do regularly.

DID YOU KNOW?

The average human heart will beat 2.5 billion times during a lifetime.

WHAT'S STOPPING YOU?

Recent studies have shown that you don't even need to exercise for a long time each day to get a benefit from it. Three bursts of 10 minutes of activity each day will help maintain a healthy heart.

Of course, you probably already know this. But do you do it – or enough of it? Most of us don't. And why? Because we think it's too hard. Or it's boring. Or we've got a sore knee or a sore back. Or we just don't have time.

If you're using any of these excuses, maybe it's time to have a talk to yourself! There is nearly always a way to get around challenges. After all, if people who have had spinal injuries can play basketball, and legally blind people can run marathons, then surely you can get out for a walk. It's actually a matter of finding something that you enjoy and finding a way to make it fit into your day.

Enjoyment is essential, because you're never going to stick with something you hate. People find enjoyment in different ways – so which is yours?

 # **Social:** Do you love getting out for adventures with your kids? Or does spending time with like-minded friends appeal more?

 # **Physical:** Is it the actual act of running/walking/cycling that you enjoy? Or is it the great feeling that you get afterwards?

 # **Challenge:** How do you feel about the idea of setting yourself a big, hairy challenge and actually achieving it?

 # **Novelty:** Are you motivated by trying new things, or seeing new places?

If you're not sure what's going to make you feel good, try some different activities and see what agrees with your head and your body. You don't have to spend a lot of money on this, either. It costs nothing to get out for a walk. If you don't have a bike, you could either buy a cheap one or see whether you can borrow one from a similarly sized friend. Swimming in the ocean is free, and it's not too expensive at a pool – chances are you'd spend more on lunch than you would on your entry fee.

Of course, that still leaves the 'sore knee/sore back/too old' issue. Well, the good news is that it's quite likely that whatever you're using as an excuse will actually be improved by activity. A lack of movement can make a dodgy joint more painful, or keep a sore back from improving. It's a long time since bed rest has been seen as the cure for a sore back. And you are never too old to do something! There are yoga instructors in their nineties, triathletes in their eighties and ultrarunners in their seventies. If you're lacking inspiration, google 'old athletes' and see if the results change your perspective.

HOW TO GET GOING

You don't have to want to run a marathon, climb a mountain, or cycle the Tour de France. Instead, you need to find a goal and activity that's right for *you*. Whatever that is, the important thing is to start out easy and build up progressively. Admit that you're not a highly tuned athlete, swallow your pride and start slowly. That way, you'll see yourself get better and better over time.

On the following pages there is a graded activity programme that you can use to build your aerobic fitness in whatever sport you choose. When you're doing these workouts, make sure that you keep the intensity at the right level. If you do your 'easy' sessions at full whack, you'll just wear yourself out and will probably have to start all over again. It's much easier to get it right the first time! There are three levels to the workouts:

1. **Easy:** This means easy! You shouldn't be puffing – you should be able to talk quite comfortably, and you should be able to do this for the entire duration of the exercise.
2. **Moderate:** Now you're puffing, but you can still hold a conversation, although it's a bit uncomfortable.
3. **Hard:** This is definitely 'work'. You're breathing hard, and conversation is difficult. There is no sign of comfort!

After you've done each workout, take a moment to reflect on it. Did you enjoy it? If not, was it *all* awful, or only part of it? What would make it more enjoyable? Taking the time to think about your workouts, your challenges and your achievements puts you in control – you become your own coach. This is something that professional athletes do. Even though they have loads of highly qualified advisors they can call on, they make sure that they're in charge of their own destiny.

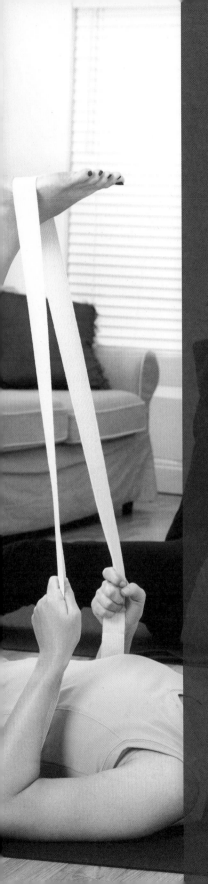

FIT:5

Muscle maintenance kit

Building muscle is one thing, but those muscles also have to be in good shape to function effectively. Looking after your muscles is easy to forget – but it's also easy to do! You don't need much equipment – these five items will be more than enough for most people:

1. A foam roller – long or short, knobbly or smooth, hollow or solid, it doesn't really matter.
2. A ball to get into muscles in awkward places – you can buy a massage ball, but a simple tennis ball is usually just as good.
3. A long resistance band or yoga strap, to help you get into some stretch positions.
4. Some massage wax, if you like to work out knots and muscle tension that way.
5. Music or a podcast to help you relax while you're helping your muscles stay healthy!

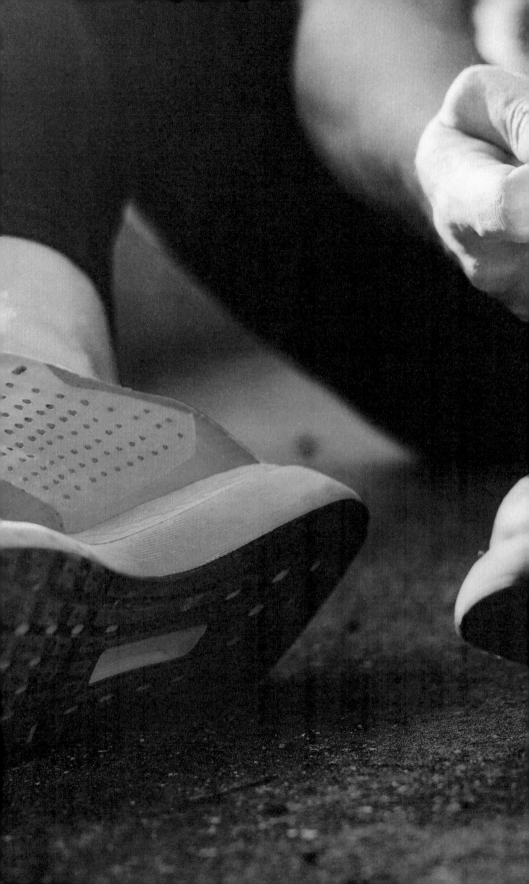

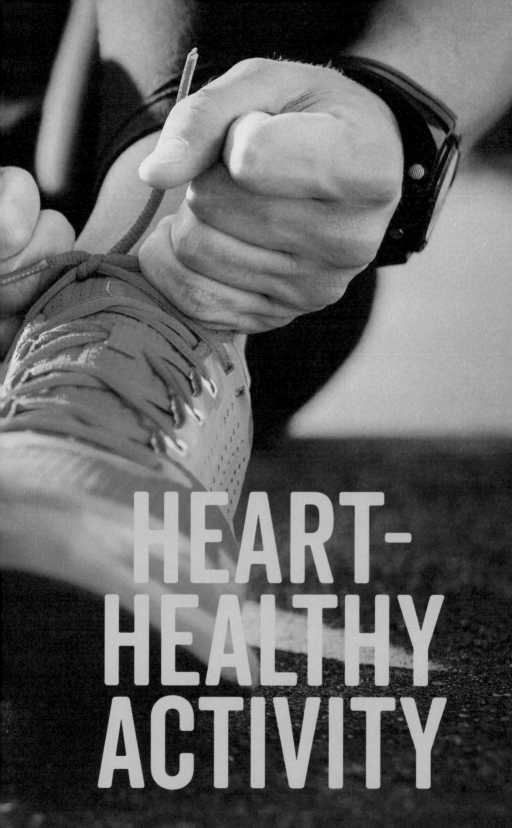

HEART-HEALTHY ACTIVITY

GO FOR YOUR GOALS

Barbara, 65

A couple of years ago I found myself in a bit of a slump. I'd had concussion and it had left its mark on me. I'd stopped running; I felt tired, overweight, undermotivated and generally fed up with myself.

I wasn't the person I used to be. I certainly didn't feel like the captain of a Boeing 777, with a lifestyle block, two adult children and a love of sailing, diving, swimming and skiing! I knew I needed to get back to who I was, and so I joined Nic's programme.

I am so glad I made this choice – it transformed my life. I ended up being extremely fit: I was running a half-marathon every couple of months, I could swim 2 km in the ocean and I was sleeping well and eating properly. Of course, this didn't happen overnight. I started running short distances every day, and recording everything that I ate. I love the apps that Nic suggests we use – MyFitnessPal and MapMyRun are my two favourites.

Another key to my success was setting small and large goals. Initially, my small goal just involved running a bit further each week; eventually I was able to add a big goal of running a half-marathon. Once I had that goal in mind and I'd built up my running distance, I started looking at races, which helped keep me motivated.

Being outside and being active made me a happier person. I ran all over my local area and got to see much more than if I had just stayed indoors or worked out in a gym. Mentally, I felt so much more positive than before I started the programme.

If you're thinking about making changes to improve your health, my advice is to get started now, even if you only make small changes. And talk to your friends about it, too – because once they see how great it is for you, they'll want to get involved as well.

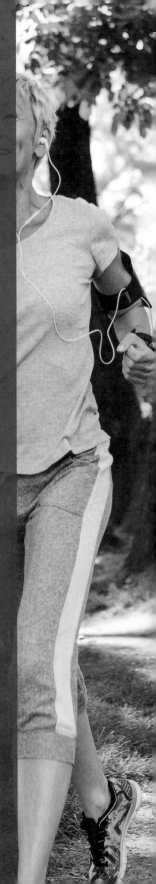

BEGINNER LEVEL

One of the most common mistakes people make when starting an exercise programme is to do too much, too soon. This nearly always ends in injury and/or disillusionment. If your activity currently consists of walking from the couch to the fridge, don't even think about starting at anywhere but this beginner level. It only lasts three months, and you'll give yourself a really solid base to build on.

Current activity level: Inactive.
Activity choice: Walk, walk/jog, jog, run, cycle, swim, cross-train, other aerobic activity.
How this works: Each week you are going to do at least two workouts (ideally three). You can choose whatever aerobic activity you like, and you can mix it up throughout the 12 weeks. The point of this is to get you moving for a set amount of time and to gradually add some intensity in to your workout.
So, the first week you might do three walk/jogs, or you might do one walk/jog, one cycle and one swim, each for 20 minutes. What you choose is entirely up to you. The 'Your Workouts' graphic overleaf shows the different workouts that you'll use; the 'Your Progression' graphic shows when to use them. Don't be tempted to skip ahead – just enjoy each workout as you do it.
After 12 weeks, you will have built up to just over 2 hours of aerobic exercise per week, and you'll be ready to move on to the intermediate programme.

YOUR WORKOUTS

A:20

20 MINS EASY

D:40

10 MINS EASY
20 MINS MODERATE
10 MINS EASY

B:25

10 MINS EASY
10 MINS MODERATE
5 MINS EASY

E:45

10 MINS EASY,
5 MINS MODERATE,
5 MINS HARD, 5 MINS EASY,
5 MINS MODERATE,
5 MINS HARD, 10 MINS EASY

C:30

10 MINS EASY
15 MINS MODERATE
5 MINS EASY

F:45

45 MINS EASY

YOUR PROGRESSION

WEEK	WORKOUT	WORKOUT	WORKOUT	TOTAL TIME (WEEK)
1	A	A	A	60 MIN
2	A	B	A	65 MIN
3	A	B	C	75 MIN
4	B	B	C	80 MIN
5	B	C	C	85 MIN
6	B	C	D	95 MIN
7	B	C	D	95 MIN
8	C	C	D	100 MIN
9	C	C	D	100 MIN
10	C	D	E	115 MIN
11	D	E	F	130 MIN
12	D	E	F	130 MIN

DON'T LISTEN
TO THE DREAM-STEALERS

Mark, 35

In my line of work, I'm lucky - or unlucky! - enough to have annual medical checks as part of the job. Each year, I'd hear the same thing - you're a bit overweight, your blood pressure's a bit high, your blood results are OK but a bit average. I'd been ignoring it, I guess, and then one day I saw a photo of myself and thought 'That's not me!'. It was the kick I needed to do something - and that something was signing up to Nic's programme.

That was two years ago, but what Nic said at those first few meetings has stuck with me. The great thing is that his message is simple and is based on science. That doesn't mean it's always easy to do, though! I cut out simple carbohydrates and made my plate more colourful, but I did feel quite flat for the first few weeks. And then after 6 weeks, it all just seemed to happen. My energy levels were so much more stable - no ups and downs. After 12 weeks, I'd lost 8 kg.

I've always been a bit competitive, and even before I started on Nic's programme I was quite into my cycling - but I was getting beaten by my friends, which I didn't like! I added in HIIT training and weight training, and the combination of that plus my new way of eating led to my skinfold reading [a body fat indicator] decreasing and my lean muscle mass increasing. As a result, I've gone from being a participant in cycling races to a competitor - I shocked some of our club members when I did the round Taupo ride in 5 hours 10 minutes, which was a massive improvement on the previous year when I took 6 hours and 50 minutes.

It's not just cycling, though. I feel very different. I'm much more confident in going about things, just day to day. I recover from challenges so much more quickly than I did before. For me, being healthy is about being able to do the things that you enjoy, physically and mentally. Being physically healthier makes me feel stronger mentally, and I know I can set myself ambitious goals and take on all sorts of challenges that I might have avoided before.

If I had to give one piece of advice to someone who was thinking about making changes for the sake of their health, I'd say do it! Don't procrastinate. Start now. Set a goal, get some supportive people around you, arm yourself with some apps to monitor your progress, be honest, and keep your eye on the long-term goal. Don't listen to the dream-stealers - show them exactly what can be done.

And if you need any more motivation, think of this: 'If you don't look after your body, where are you going to live when you're older?'

INTERMEDIATE LEVEL

Once you have achieved a moderate level of activity, you can look to increase your effort a bit. What's moderate? It's exercising regularly, two to three times a week, for 20–30 minutes at a time. If you complete the beginner programme, you'll fit into this category nicely.

Current activity level: Somewhat active.
Activity choice: Walk, walk/jog, jog, run, cycle, swim, cross-train, other aerobic activity.
How this works: Each week you are going to do three workouts. Ideally most of these will be the same type of aerobic exercise, but you can mix it up throughout the 12 weeks.
The point of this plan is to build both the duration and the intensity of the exercise that you're doing. The 'Your Workouts' graphic overleaf shows the different workouts you'll use; the 'Your Progression' graphic shows when to use them. Don't be tempted to skip ahead – just enjoy each workout as you do it.
After 12 weeks, you will have built up to two and a half hours of aerobic exercise per week, and you'll be ready to move on to the advanced programme, if you feel like attempting it.

A:30
30 MINS EASY

D:50
10 MINS EASY
10 MINS MODERATE
10 MINS HARD
10 MINS MODERATE
10 MINS EASY

B:35
10 MINS EASY
15 MINS MODERATE
10 MINS EASY

E:50
10 MINS EASY, 5 MINS MODERATE,
5 MINS EASY, 5 MINS HARD
5 MINS EASY, 5 MINS HARD
5 MINS EASY, 5 MINS HARD
5 MINS EASY

C:40
10 MINS EASY
20 MINS MODERATE
10 MINS EASY

F:50
50 MINS EASY

YOUR PROGRESSION

WEEK	WORKOUT 1	WORKOUT 2	WORKOUT 2	TOTAL TIME FOR THE WEEK
1	A	A	A	90 MIN
2	A	B	A	95 MIN
3	A	B	C	105 MIN
4	B	B	C	110 MIN
5	B	C	C	115 MIN
6	B	C	D	125 MIN
7	B	C	D	125 MIN
8	C	C	D	130 MIN
9	C	C	D	130 MIN
10	C	D	E	140 MIN
11	D	E	F	150 MIN
12	D	E	F	150 MIN

GRAB THE EASY CHANGES

Kevin, 61

A combination of getting older and having a slack winter meant that I'd gained way too much weight – and worse, I'd lost a lot of muscle mass. My shirt size was 3XL, my trousers were nearly too small and my BMI showed that I was getting close to morbidly obese. I do not want to get to retirement and find that I'm too unhealthy to enjoy it, so I knew I had to do something. Luckily, we have a wellness programme at work and through that I got the opportunity to join Nic's programme.

I was pretty surprised when he suggested bacon for breakfast instead of toast, but I gave it a go, having an egg and two slices of bacon instead of my usual egg and two slices of toast. I got rid of the carbs and junk food that I used to have for dinner, and got stuck into chicken salad instead. Chicken salad became my friend!

I increased my exercise, adding in more walking and some strength work. This was really helped by our situation at work – we have a big site and we constructed a walkway around it, with exercise stations along the way. It didn't cost much as we did it ourselves, and used recycled materials and built it bit by bit. We've got yoga mats and chin-up bars, a lunge lane and a balance beam, and a 'stairway to heaven' to get the heart rate up. Loads of people use it, including me. It's so easy because it's right on site.

All of these small changes have made a big difference: I've dropped a pants size and my breathing is much better. In early 2018 I walked around Lake Rotorua – that's 43.6 km. There's no way I could have done that before.

If someone asks me for advice about being more healthy, I say go for the easy changes. Lose the milk and sugar from your tea; park further from the door. All those little changes are sustainable, and that's what will make you successful. Oh, and learn to enjoy the feeling of hunger – think of it as an accomplishment, not a problem!

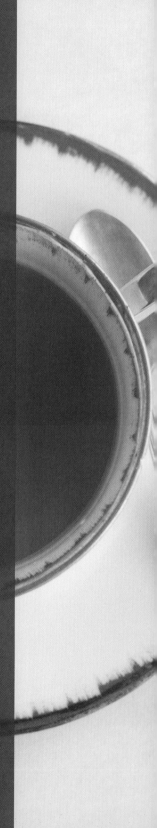

ADVANCED LEVEL

If you decide that you want to get really serious about your aerobic fitness, then you can progress to the advanced level. This would be a great thing to do if you decided you wanted to tackle a half-marathon or a triathlon or a distance swim – whatever gets you going. This isn't a training programme for any of those events, but it will give you a solid base to start from.

- # **Current activity level:** Active.
- # **Activity choice:** Walk, walk/jog, run, cycle, swim, cross-train, other aerobic activity.
- # **How this works:** Each week you are going to do three workouts. Ideally most of these will be the same type of aerobic exercise, but you can mix it up throughout the 12 weeks.
- # The point of this plan is to build both the duration and the intensity of the exercise that you're doing. The 'Your Workouts' graphic overleaf shows the different workouts that you'll use; the 'Your Progression' graphic shows when to use them. Don't be tempted to skip ahead – just enjoy each workout as you do it.
- # After 12 weeks, you will have built up to nearly 3 hours of aerobic exercise per week, and you'll have a solid base of fitness that will contribute to your general health as well as set you up for any sporting challenges you want to take on.

A:30

30 MINS EASY

D:50

10 MINS EASY, 5 MINS MODERATE
5 MINS HARD, 5 MINS EASY
5 MINS MODERATE, 5 MINS HARD,
5 MINS EASY, 5 MINS MODERATE
5 MINS EASY

B:40

10 MINS EASY
20 MINS MODERATE
10 MINS EASY

E:60

10 MINS EASY, 10 MINS MODERATE,
5 MINS HARD, 5 MINS EASY
5 MINS HARD, 5 MINS EASY
5 MINS HARD, 5 MINS EASY
5 MINS MODERATE, 5 MINS EASY

C:45

10 MINS EASY
10 MINS MODERATE
5 MINS HARD, 5 MINS EASY
10 MINS MODERATE
5 MINS EASY

F:60

60 MINS EASY

YOUR PROGRESSION

WEEK	WORKOUT 1	WORKOUT 2	WORKOUT 3	TOTAL TIME FOR THE WEEK
1	A	A	A	90 MIN
2	A	B	A	100 MIN
3	A	B	C	115 MIN
4	B	B	C	125 MIN
5	B	C	C	130 MIN
6	B	C	D	135 MIN
7	B	C	D	135 MIN
8	C	C	D	140 MIN
9	C	C	D	140 MIN
10	C	D	E	155 MIN
11	D	E	F	170 MIN
12	D	E	F	170 MIN

#12 MAKE THE CONNECTION

WHAT YOUR BODY DOES

Muscles and bones need something to connect them together. Your muscles are connected to your bones by tendons, and your bones are connected to other bones by ligaments. Tendons and ligaments are very similar. They're both made up largely of a protein called collagen, they don't have much in the way of blood supply, and they are much less stretchy than your muscles.

Ligaments hold your skeleton together and help to make your joints stable. If your ligaments are very lax (loose), then you're likely to have a large range of motion – you might be able to put your leg behind your head, or do something equally weird and impressive! Ligaments aren't as strong as tendons, and it's relatively easy to damage them in high-impact sports. A good example is the ACL, or anterior cruciate ligament (one of four ligaments that hold your knee together). It's quite common for this to be injured in fast-moving sports like netball and rugby.

Tendons provide a continuous connection between your muscles and your bones. They act like an energy storage unit, which helps with movement. For example, the Achilles tendon – which runs from your heel right up into your calf – works like a spring to help to propel your body forward when you're running or walking. Tendons also transmit forces from your muscles to your bones, which helps with the mechanics of movement and stops your muscles from getting exhausted! Although they're quite elastic, tendons can also get injured, with damage usually occurring where the tendon and the muscle merge into each other.

WHAT YOU CAN DO

Getting a tendon or ligament injury when you're working on your health and fitness is really annoying, especially as these injuries tend to take a long time to heal. You can't totally prevent these injuries, but you can minimise the chances of getting one by treating your connective tissue well.

YOU CAN EAT WELL

A healthy diet definitely helps – if you're eating foods that are good for your bones and muscles, then you'll be looking after your tendons and ligaments at the same time.

YOU CAN GET STRONG

A strong body also protects your connective tissue. Strong muscles help to stabilise your joints, which means that your ligaments and tendons don't need to do more work than they're designed for, and so are less likely to be overstretched or torn. It also helps if you can maintain good muscle balance, because that helps keep everything tracking in line and pulling in the right direction. Incorporating multi-joint functional exercises into your routine can help you develop good muscle balance (see page 244).

At the same time, it's important not to totally overdo things, especially when you start an exercise programme – if your muscles aren't strong enough to cope with the load you put on them, you could damage either them or their tendons. Weak muscles also mean that ligaments have to work harder to control joint movement, which puts them at greater risk of injury.

YOU CAN BE FLEXIBLE

As well as strength, having a good range of motion will benefit your tendons and ligaments. We are all born with a fantastic range of motion – just watch a baby for a few minutes, and see how flexible they are! Even as toddlers we are still able to put our joints through a huge range of motion. By the time we're teenagers, however, most of this flexibility has gone. Why? Mainly because we stop using our body this way. Instead of squatting to use a potty, we sit on a toilet. Instead of squatting to play, we sit in chair, on a couch, in a car.

This is a huge – and largely unrecognised – problem in today's society. If you stop putting your body through its full range of movement, as most of us do, your posterior chain (the muscles running down the back of your body) becomes weak and inactive. Your hamstrings become weak and super-tight; your glutes become weak and inactive – they simply stop firing and just go to sleep. As a result, you have a massive muscle imbalance, and that often leads to one of the most common health complaints around – a sore or stiff lower back.

Luckily, it is possible to reverse these effects by focusing on mobility and flexibility. Stretching lengthens a muscle, which reduces the stress on the tendons. It's not just the closest tendons that are affected, either. When a muscle is tight in one part of the body, the effect can transmit through the tissues and show up somewhere else. For example, a tight left shoulder can pull on the back muscles, which in turn can affect the right hip – and that could even cause a problem in the knee or ankle. It isn't a one-way street, either – an unstable ankle or knee can cause a sore back or a painful hip.

The great thing is that stretching and mobility exercises are easy to do – you don't need any special equipment, and you can even do it while you're watching TV. Take a look at the 'Fit 5 – Morning mobility' panel on page 85 for a basic sequence that will help keep your joints healthy, and check out the 'Mobility moves' section on page 84 for more ways to keep your body in tip-top condition.

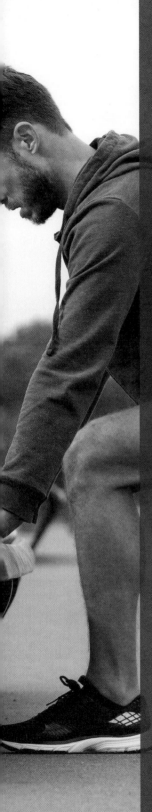

MOBILITY VERSUS FLEXIBILITY

Mobility and flexibility are both important for maintaining or improving your body's health. They are often seen as the same thing, but there is a subtle difference between the two.

Mobility is the functional movement of your body – it reflects the range of motion of your joints. If you have a bone spur in your hip, then that will restrict the range of motion of your leg. You will have less mobility in that leg as a result, so functional movements like walking and running will be impaired.

Flexibility is the isolated movement of a particular muscle complex. It's dictated by the muscle, tendons and nerves that are associated with that muscle. If you can't touch your toes, for example, this could be because your muscle/tendon complex is tight, or it could be that your sciatic nerve is trapped and hampering your flexibility.

You don't need to be flexible enough to wrap your leg around your neck, or even to grasp your hands behind your back, but the more you can improve your movement patterns, the more likely you are to stay free of injury, aches and pains. Everyone feels tight or stiff and sore in different places – once you are aware of your hot spots, you can target them so that they don't develop into a long-term problem.

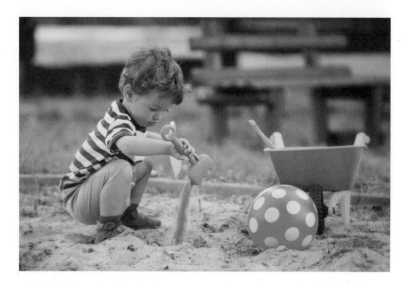

SQUAT FOR LIFE

If you've ever watched a toddler intently inspecting something in the dirt, you'll have noticed how easily they squat. Their hips are low – down below their knees; their back is straight; and they have no trouble at all maintaining this stance.

Now think about the last time you were in this position. If you're like most of us, it's probably when you were about two years old! In the Western world, as soon as we're toilet-trained we stop squatting. We sit on chairs – to eat, to work, to relax. We sit in cars, trains and planes. We sit for hours on end, year after year after year. And then, at some point, we realise that we have a sore back, or sore hips or knees or ankles. Something almost inevitably lets go.

Why? Because all that sitting reduces our range of motion. We get tight hip flexors, tight back muscles and a weak core. We effectively chop our body off in the middle, so we don't have a full-length connection from head to heel. It gets worse – as we stand up from a sitting position, we start using the wrong muscles. Instead of using our glutes and quads to drive us up, we start to use our back muscles to pull us up – and that's really not their job! No wonder back pain is such a common complaint.

You might be thinking that it's all very well for a two-year-old to squat – they're pretty close to the ground to start with – but it's not very practical for an adult. But take a look at photos from countries where office jobs and plush couches and comfortable cafés aren't quite so common. You'll see adults squatting quite naturally, so clearly it's not a movement just for kids!

Introducing deep squat movements into your daily activities will help you avoid developing chronic lower back pain, minimise the chance of you getting injuries, and prevent difficulties with running or walking. If you're relatively young, you might not think that squatting is going to make much difference to you – but it almost invariably will. Start squatting now, and you'll be so much better off when you're older. (Refer to the squat photos on page 282 to ensure your form is correct.)

Like any exercise, good form is important.

Start with your feet apart, a bit further than shoulder width. Lightly engage your core muscles, so that your back is in a neutral position, your ribs are stable and your shoulders are relaxed but square.

Squeeze your glutes, then push your bottom back – but don't let your lower back move out of neutral. As you do this, push your knees out and keep your feet firmly glued to the ground. Lower yourself down, reaching your arms forward as a counterbalance. If you find your back moving out of neutral, you're probably trying to go too deep, too soon. Ease off, because you won't be doing yourself any good.

If you're lacking range of movement in your ankles, put a book or two under your heels and hold on to something for stability.

To rise from the squat, push up using the power in your glutes.

The more time you spend squatting with good form, the sooner you'll improve your range of motion.

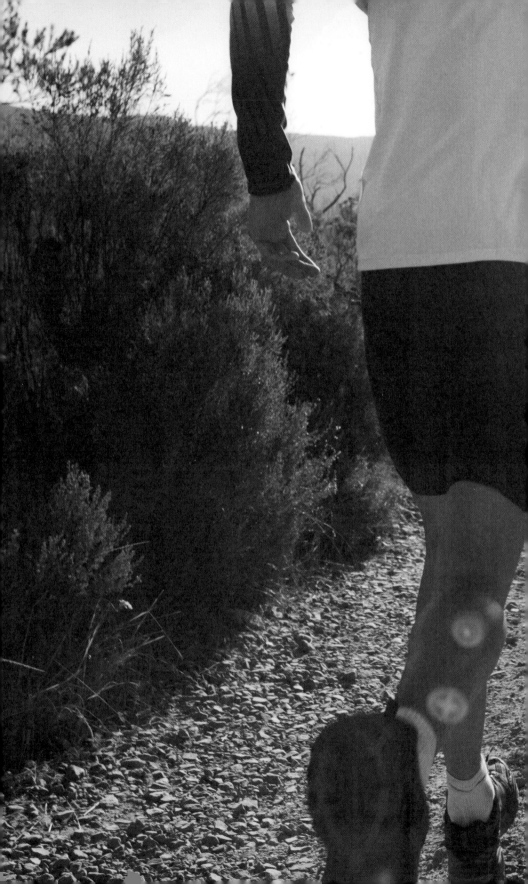

MOBILITY
MOVES

MOBILITY MOVES

Mobility moves will help to keep all the joints in your body moving smoothly and in the way they were designed to. When you're doing these exercises, don't push into pain – it's not meant to hurt. Pain means you're either trying to go beyond what your body's currently capable of doing, or your form's not right – you might be using the wrong muscles. However, the exercises might feel uncomfortable – which is fine. There's a difference between pain and discomfort!

Each time you do these, note how far you can move before things feel tight – over time, you'll see your body become increasingly supple. Don't stop once you've gained this mobility, though. You need to keep using this range of motion in order to retain it. As you work through these exercises you'll discover which are your go-to ones, the ones that you need to do regularly to help you move better and feel better.

When you do these exercises, keep these basic pointers in mind:

Breathe: Breathe evenly and calmly throughout the stretch. People often forget to breathe when they're focusing on a new exercise – and that's not a good thing.

Stabilise: Keep your core muscles lightly engaged when you're stretching, so that your body is stable. Keep it light: don't go for an all-out squeeze of your core muscles – it won't deliver any benefit and just distracts from the stretch that you're supposed to be doing.

Focus: Maintain your attention on the muscles or joints that you are working. This will help you keep good form and get the most out of the stretch. As a bonus, it makes it easier to notice your improvements over time.

Activation: Try to contract the muscle or side that is opposite the one you are stretching. For example, if you are stretching your hip flexors, squeeze your glutes so they are switched on.

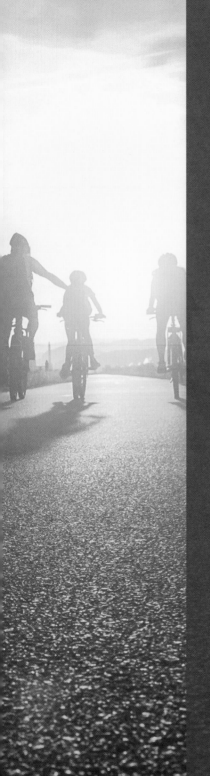

FIT:5

Morning mobility

This 10-minute routine is something you can do first thing in the morning to wake up your body. Spend a total of 2 minutes on each exercise – that's 1 minute each side for most of the exercises.

1. Cat–cow lumbar spine mobiliser (page 93)
2. Kneeling dorsiflexion to mobilise your ankle and calf (page 100)
3. Hamstring stretch (against a doorway or using a yoga strap or resistance band) (page 98)
4. Thoracic spine mobiliser – 1 minute rolling and 1 minute chest opener (pages 90, 92)
5. Couch stretch for quads and hips (page 95)

NECK MOBILITY

These exercises are great for people who spend a lot of time looking forward at a computer screen all day. They help to restore the range of motion in your neck. Poor neck mobility can lead to pain and bad posture, which will lead to more pain. Ward this off by keeping your neck in good health.

NECK ROLL

Find a small, soft ball that will raise your head off the ground but still leave your neck in neutral – you don't want your head to be tilted forwards. Lie down on your back, with your knees bent and your feet flat on the floor and place the ball under your neck.

Slowly rotate your head from side to side, pausing briefly when you get to the end of your range of motion. Repeat so that you rotate to each side 10 times.

If you find this difficult to do with a ball, try using a book or something of similar thickness that will give you more stability.

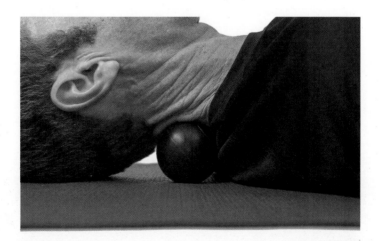

NECK STRETCH

Stand comfortably with your left arm hanging straight down beside your body. Reach your right arm around behind your back and grasp your left elbow. The back of your right wrist should be touching your back.
Now tilt your head to bring your left ear towards your left shoulder. You should feel the stretch through your right trapezius, between the base of your neck and your shoulder. Hold for 30 seconds.
Repeat on the other side with your left hand grasping your right elbow and tilting your right ear towards your right shoulder.

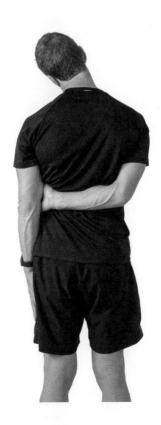

NODDING DOG

\# Standing or sitting with good posture, slowly bend your head forward (flexion) to look at the floor, then up and back to look at the ceiling (extension). Make sure the movement comes from your neck, not from your back – don't let your back or shoulders hunch over when you're moving.

\# Repeat so that you do 10–20 full movements.

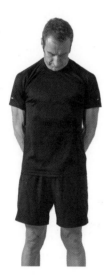
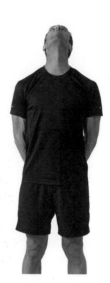

ROLL IT OUT

Technically called self-myofascial release, foam rolling is a great way to give your body a massage. You can work on trigger points, knots and adhesions, all of which will respond to pressure and movement. As you roll, you are stretching out your tissues and this can help increase your mobility. Getting stuck into tight spots can help relax muscles, which again benefits your mobility.

Foam rolling is simple – just roll your body slowly over the roller, and stop on any spot that feels tender. Stay on the muscle and stay off your tendons, though. Do the same with a ball, but use it to get into smaller, more awkward spots. Treat these parts of your body to a foam roll on a regular basis:

1. Glutes - Use a roller or a ball, whichever is easiest. Be careful not to crush the tendons around your sit bones – stay in the meaty part of your glutes.
2. Calves - Go slowly; take 5-10 seconds to roll the length of your calf. Go down the outside and inside, as well as down the middle. If you find a particularly sore spot, try pulsing back and forwards over it.
3. Thoracic spine - Ideally, get hold of a little peanut massage ball; they are fairly cheap and are great for rolling out the muscles either side of your spine. You can also use a standard foam roller or one with a central groove that your spine fits into. If you don't have these, try standing with your back to the wall and using a tennis ball to roll up and down your spinal muscles.
4. Quads - A foam roller is perfect for your quads. Roll the outside, inside and centre parts of the muscles, and if you need to, increase the weight by stacking one leg on top of the other.
5. Foot - The plantar fascia is the tissue on the base of your foot, and it will really benefit from a good roll with a tennis ball. This is pretty painful for a lot of people when they first start out – which means that the tissue really needs this work! Persevere, but don't put yourself into too much distress. After a couple of weeks, you'll notice that it doesn't hurt so much.

SPINE AND CHEST MOBILITY

These are great exercises for everyone! They help to counteract the forward hunch that we often develop after spending so much time sitting in cars, at desks and on the sofa.

SPINE ROLL

- \# Position a foam roller under your back, starting with it up by your shoulders. Gently support your head with your hands.
- \# Breathe in; then, as you breathe out, let your head and upper body relax back into the stretch.
- \# Lift up slightly as you breathe in, and roll a bit further down the roller – just go down one vertebra at a time. Again, breathe out and relax.
- \# Repeat until the roller is down near your lumbar spine/ lower back.
- \# If you want to really get into the muscles that run down either side of your spine, get a peanut massage ball (or build a DIY version by taping two tennis balls together). Rolling on this helps to target the muscles without the rest of your back spreading the load.

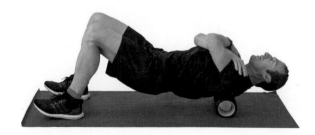

BOOK OPENER

Lie on your side, on the floor (you need a firm surface
    underneath you). Keeping a straight line down through
    your back, bend your knees and put both arms out in
    front of you, one on top of the other.
Lift the top arm and, as you do this, rotate your upper
    body, bringing your arm up and over so that it lies flat on
    the ground. Your hips should not move.
Reverse the movement to come back to the starting
    position.
Do 10 book openers on each side.

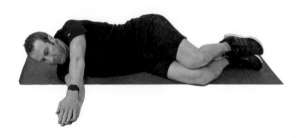

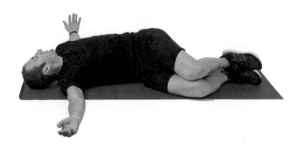

CHEST OPENER

\# Take a yoga strap or a towel and hold it in front of you, with your arms spread wide.

\# Raise your arms up to bring the towel over the top of your head, and continue to rotate your shoulders so that the towel ends up behind your head. You'll find a place where the stretch is strongest; hold it there for about 30 seconds.

\# Bring the towel back to the front and repeat.

\# If you don't feel a stretch, bring your hands closer together by 1 centimetre and try again.

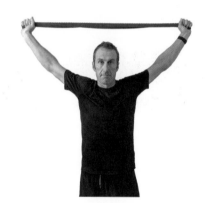

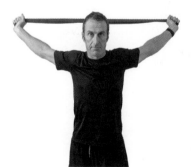
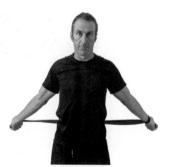

CAT-COW

Kneel on all fours, hands under your shoulders, knees under your hips, head in a straight line with your spine, back in neutral.

Breathe in and sink your abdomen towards the ground, at the same time moving your tailbone and head up towards the sky. The shape from your head to your tailbone should look like a skatebowl – or a cow with a saggy backbone!

Breathe out and reverse the motion, rotating your pelvis so that your back arches, and rolling your head forward so you are looking down at the floor. The shape of your back should resemble a cat that's got a fright! This movement feels great if you do it slowly, moving just one vertebra at a time. In the cat position, push your hands down into the floor to get the most out of the stretch, and let your head hang so you're not tightening up your neck muscles.

Repeat for as many times as feels good!

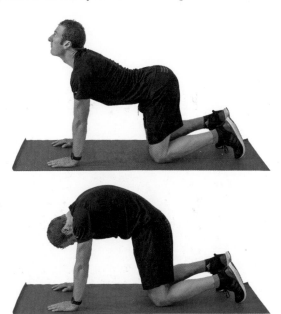

HIP MOBILITY

Sitting all day makes our hip flexors tighten up, which in turn makes it hard to stand up straight or get down into a squat. These mobility exercises are great for the hips – they help improve overall hip function, so that you can walk, run and play with ease. If you've ever stood up and felt really stiff down the front of your hips, then these are definitely exercises you need to do.

COWBOY LUNGE

Rotating your body in this exercise helps to mobilise your hips in all directions: too often we just focus on the front-back aspect of a movement, forgetting that our body moves – or should move! – much more widely than this.

- # Kneel on your left knee, right foot flat on the floor in front of you. Push forward with your hips, to feel a stretch down the front of your left leg.
- # Hold for 30 seconds, then ramp it up by rotating your upper body towards your right leg.
- # Hold for another 30 seconds, then put your right hand on your right knee and push away from you, while at the same time rotating your upper body to the left. Put your left hand on the floor to stabilise yourself and deepen the stretch. Hold for 30 seconds.
- # Repeat on the other side.

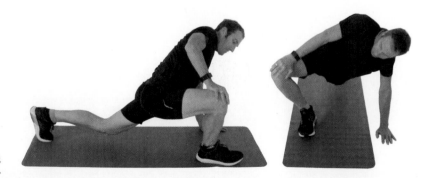

COUCH STRETCH

\# Start by kneeling close to a wall, stool or in front of a couch, facing away from it. If you're kneeling on a hard surface, put a cushion or some padding on the ground to protect your knees.

\# Put your right leg out in front of you, with your calf vertical. Put your left leg behind you, with your knee on the ground and your foot on the wall or couch. If you're tight through your quads or hip flexors, you might not be able to get your left calf vertical.

\# Lean forward and put both hands on the floor. Squeeze your right glute and push your right hip towards the ground. Hold for 30–60 seconds. You'll feel the stretch in your left quad and/or left hip, but the adductors on your right leg will get a workout as well.

\# If this gets easy, then straighten your body, which will increase the stretch through your quads and hip flexors. Most people will struggle to do this. It's best to progress to this position slowly, using a low chair or stool to hold on to until you are able to fully raise your body and keep your left glute switched on the entire time.

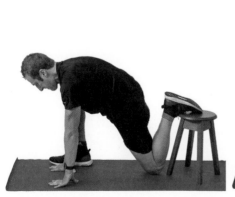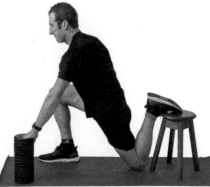

PIGEON

The key to getting good results from this exercise is keeping your bent leg at 90 degrees – if you let your foot drift in towards your body, you'll decrease the effectiveness of the stretch. If you find this really challenging, start with a cushion under the thigh of your front leg and then discard it once you have built up more flexibility.

Kneel on the ground and place your right leg in front of you, bent at the knee so that your lower leg is at a 90-degree angle to your thigh. Your left leg should be stretched out behind you – aim to get it straight behind you, rather than drifting out to the side.

Support yourself with your hands on the ground in front of your right leg, and sink into the stretch; hold for 30 seconds.

Walk your hands to the right to change the angle of the stretch and hold for another 30 seconds, then move your hands to the left and hold once more.

Repeat on the other side.

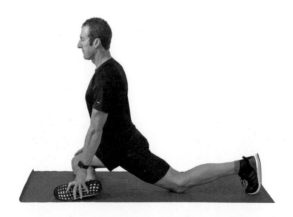

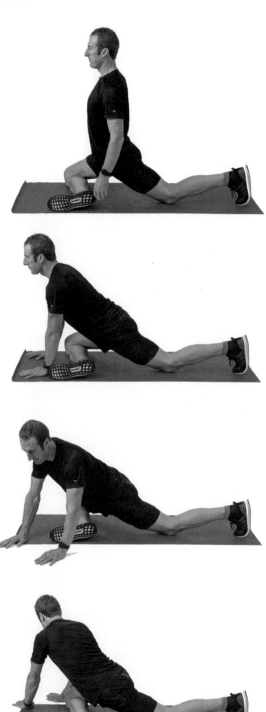

HAMSTRING FLEXIBILITY

Our hamstrings tend to get under-used these days, thanks to our limited range of hip motion and the fact that we don't squat much any more. Still, they're vital for a healthy gait, whether you're walking or running. These exercises will help to keep them healthy. The exercises are listed from easiest to most challenging: start out by doing the easiest one, then replace it with a harder one as you gain mobility, stability and strength.

STRAIGHT LEG RAISE

Lie on your back, your legs out straight in front of you.
Keeping the leg straight, raise your right leg as high as you can, maintaining control throughout the lift. Then lower it with control.
Repeat 10 times on each leg. The movement is a controlled raise, not a kick.

STRAIGHT LEG STRETCH

Lie on your back close to a wall with a corner, or in a doorway (preferably one where you're not going to get trampled on by people walking through!).
Place your right leg up on the wall; your left leg will be flat on the ground in front of you (which is why you need a corner or a doorway, otherwise that leg's got nowhere to go). Inch your body closer to the wall to get a good stretch through your hamstrings. Hold for 30 seconds, then repeat on the other side.

CONE PICK-UP

Also known as the single-leg Romanian deadlift, this exercise will challenge your balance as well as your hamstring function. This is a variation on the exercise described on page 273. This is a very powerful, functional exercise with strength and stretch components. If you do one version, then you can leave the other version out of your routine.

Stand on your right leg with the knee slightly flexed. Engage your glutes and your core, then pivot forward at the hips, lifting your left leg up behind you, so that your body is parallel to the ground. Imagine that you are going to pick up a cone that's on the ground in front of you.

Use your hamstrings to pull your body back upright – don't drag yourself up with your back muscles. You can actually put a cone or similar object in front of you and pick it up, if you like – but don't add weight until you have really mastered this exercise.

Repeat 10 times on one side, then do the same on the other side.

Add a bit of variation by turning this into a walking exercise, alternating sides and swinging through to take a step each time you return to the vertical.

ANKLE MOBILITY

Spending all day in shoes – especially ones with raised heels – and walking on even surfaces robs us of the natural flexibility of our ankles. When your heel is raised all the time, your Achilles tendons and calf muscles shorten, and that reduces your ankle's range of motion, which in turn affects your ability to squat, and use your glutes, hips, hamstrings and core. These exercises will help to restore that, improving your ability to squat as well as your overall mobility.

STEP STRETCH

Stand on one leg on a step, so that your heel is unsupported. Ease your weight back so that you feel a stretch down through your Achilles tendon and lower calf.
Hold for 30 seconds, then repeat on the other side.

WALL STRETCH

Face a wall and, with the heel of your right foot on the ground, place the toes of that foot against the wall. Lean forwards to create a stretch down the back of your lower calf.
Hold for 30 seconds, then repeat on the other side.

KNEELING DORSIFLEXION

Kneel on your right knee, with your right foot flat on the floor and your leg tucked back as far as it will go.

\# Gently move your weight forward, so that you are working the right ankle muscles, tendons and ligaments. Roll your weight forward and back, and then side to side.

\# Work on each foot for about 1–2 minutes.

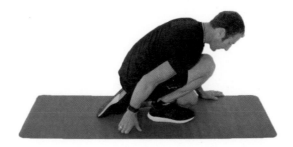

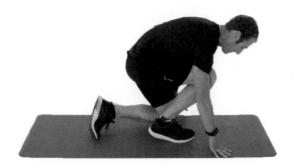

#13 TIME OUT!

If just reading about all of those exercises has left you exhausted, don't panic. You don't have to do them all. Think of the exercise options as a menu – you choose what you want each day. Some days you might just want to do a bit of mobility work; other days, it might be strength training. It depends on your lifestyle and goals.

If you want to improve your health, the key is to do a bit more activity than you have been doing in the past. If that's just an extra 10 minutes each day, or 30 minutes three days a week, that's fine – as long as it's more than you have been doing and as long as it's challenging you. Here are some examples of how you could slowly work your way into an exercise habit, or build on your existing activity levels.

ABSOLUTE NEWBIE

If you've never exercised before or if it's been a while since you've done anything like this, then try this simple 10-week programme to start your journey to health.

Week 1: Commit to three 20-minute sessions of aerobic exercise (brisk walk, bike, swim).

Week 2: Add in one body maintenance session (foam rolling or self-massage). Allow 20 minutes for this.

Week 3: Add in one strength session (just five exercises from the functional exercises on pages 244 to 293). Allow 30 minutes for this. If repeating the exercises three times is too challenging, do fewer reps or sets, but aim to increase this later on.

Week 4: Add in a mobility session (just five exercises from the mobility moves on pages 84 to 101). Allow 20 minutes for this.

Week 5: Add in a second foam rolling session.

Week 6: Add in a second strength session.

Week 7: Add in a second mobility session.

Week 8: Increase the duration of your aerobic exercise to 30 minutes each time.

Week 9: Add in a third strength session.

Week 10: Add in a third mobility session.

Remember, some of this can be done while you are watching TV – you don't even have to leave the lounge!

ERRATIC EXERCISER

If your problem is not so much with doing exercise, but with having a structured plan, then see if you can build a week that works for you.

Day 1
 # Aerobic exercise (the type and duration will depend on what you're currently doing).
 # Body maintenance session.

Day 2
 # Strength session – choose five exercises from the functional exercises on pages 244 to 293 and do three sets of each.
 # Mobility session – choose one exercise from each of the mobility moves on pages 84 to 101. If you know you've got a problem area, spend a bit more time on that.

Day 3
 # Aerobic exercise.
 # Body maintenance session.

Day 4
 # Strength session.
 # Mobility session.

Day 5
 # Aerobic exercise.
 # Body maintenance session.

Day 6
 # Strength session.
 # Mobility session.

Day 7
 # Body maintenance session or day off.

Remember, body maintenance can be done while you're watching TV in the evening. You can even do your mobility sessions in front of the TV if you like, as long as you remain focused on what you're doing, and not what's happening on screen. On days when you have two activities scheduled, feel free to split them up so you do one in the morning and one in the evening. Make it work for you.

TOTALLY TIME CHALLENGED

We all have those days when time just gets sucked away in the vortex of life and there is absolutely no way you can get out for a 30-minute walk, or spend 45 minutes strength training. However, those days do not have to be a total loss – you can still get in a short burst of activity that will get your heart pumping and build strength at the same time. This is the '10-minute kicker' programme – think of it as your own personal emergency kit that will stop you losing fitness when life gets in the way.

The rules
- # Set a timer for 10 minutes.
- # Make sure to keep perfect form when doing the exercises.
- # Transition between exercises quickly – don't be tempted to take a breather!

Option A
- # Choose five exercises from the functional fitness list on pages 244 to 293.
- # Perform each exercise for 30 seconds.
- # Repeat this four times, which makes a total of 10 minutes.

Option B
- # Choose five exercises from the functional fitness list on pages 244 to 293.
- # Perform 10 reps of each exercise, then move to the next one.
- # Keep repeating this '10 reps by 5 exercise' pattern until you have done a total of 10 minutes.

Option C

Choose 10 exercises from the functional fitness list on pages 244 to 293.

Perform each exercise for 30 seconds.

Repeat this twice, which makes a total of 10 minutes.

Option D

Choose five exercises from the functional fitness list on pages 244 to 293.

Perform 20 reps of each exercise, then move to the next one.

Keep repeating this '20 reps by 5 exercise' pattern until you have done a total of 10 minutes.

#14 PROTECTION AND PADDING

WHAT YOUR BODY DOES

Fat – now that's a word that can make health-conscious people squirm. But we all have fat in our bodies, and it's really important that we do. Fat – or adipose tissue, to give it its more scientific name – is essential for maintaining a healthy body. It surrounds some of our organs, helping to protect them against damage from bumps and bashes. It sits in an insulating layer under our skin, keeping us warm when temperatures fall. And it stores energy so that we can survive when food supplies become low. There are two types of fat in our bodies – white and brown.

White fat is regarded as the less desirable form: this is the type of fat that increases when we put on weight. It's where all of our excess energy (which comes from eating too much food) is stored. White fat especially accumulates around the waist. Each cell of white fat has one big globule of fat in it, taking up about 90% of the available space. Even though it's mainly fat, white fat tissue is still quite metabolically active. It produces various substances that are involved in inflammation. Some of these substances promote insulin resistance and high blood pressure, among other health problems. There's strong evidence that as we get more and more excess white fat, this leads to a rollercoaster of metabolic change that makes us much more likely to develop type 2 diabetes and/or metabolic syndrome.

Brown fat is seen as much more desirable. Brown fat actually burns energy, generating heat in the process. It can do this because it contains lots of mitochondria, the cell's power-plants that burn glucose and fatty acids to produce energy. Levels of brown fat are relatively high in

children – which might explain why they're quite happy to run around in the cold with virtually no clothes on! Adults have brown fat too, but much less of it.

Imagine that you had too much white fat, but you could turn some of it into brown fat. Well, scientific research is just starting to show that this could actually be possible. Scattered through your white fat tissue are beige fat cells, and under the right conditions these cells can convert white fat cells into brown fat cells. There's now a lot of research looking at how this process could be triggered, especially by drugs – a pharmaceutical company that could come up with something that would help white fat turn into brown would be onto a winner! However, all of the current research has been done either in tissue cultures or with mice. It will probably be a long time before we see any outcomes that are relevant for people.

YOUR BODY IS OUT TO GET YOU

We humans probably store more than the bare minimum of fat as a result of evolutionary success. Thousands of years ago, if food was scarce then those people who had more fat reserves would be more likely to survive and reproduce, passing their fat-storage abilities on to their children.

Today, for many of us, food is never far away. This means that if we eat more than we need, our fat-storage system kicks in and tucks away the excess energy in our cells, rather than burning it off as heat. The outcome for most of us is unwanted weight gain that in no way promotes our long-term survival.

One thing that does seem clear, though, is that cold encourages some white fat cells to change to brown ones. Again, this has only been shown to happen in mice, but there doesn't seem to be any reason why it shouldn't also apply to us. Obviously, extreme cold won't do you any good – you'd be more likely to get frostbite than brown fat. But turning the heating down a degree or two at home or in the office might just be enough to turn a few fat-storage cells into fat-burning ones.

LOCATION, LOCATION, LOCATION

So, we all have fat in our bodies, and it's essential to have *some*. Just to function, men need to have a minimum of 2–4% body fat and women need 10–12%. Someone who's fit but not a professional athlete will probably have 14–17% fat if they're a man and 21–24% if they're a woman. An obese man is likely to have at least 26% of his bodyweight as fat; his female counterpart will have at least 32% of her bodyweight as fat. Today, it's becoming increasingly common to see people who have half of their bodyweight as fat. That's staggering, and it's definitely not healthy.

The fat that you *do* need is called essential fat. It's found in bone marrow, muscles, the brain and some organs – for instance, some sits over your kidneys to protect them. When you start to lose your essential fat – perhaps because of serious illness – your body starts to malfunction.

The rest of the fat that you carry is called non-essential fat, and this comes in two flavours – subcutaneous fat and visceral fat. They're the same type of fat, but they have different effects because of their location.

DID YOU KNOW?

A person who is not overweight still has between 30 billion and 50 billion fat cells in their body.

Subcutaneous fat is stored below the surface of the skin. It's the fat you can pinch just about anywhere on your body. This is your long-term energy store – in the event of a famine, you can start using up this fat and it will keep you going until food becomes more plentiful. While having a lot of subcutaneous fat isn't exactly good for you, it doesn't do as much harm as visceral fat.

Visceral fat is stored throughout the body. The visceral region is the central part of your body – basically the internal organs of your chest and abdomen. Visceral fat is stored in your liver, pancreas, heart and blood vessels – and because these organs are not designed to store fat, you can end up with problems if you have too much there.

Exactly *how* visceral fat causes health problems is still under investigation, but the latest research indicates that there are two main types of effect – local and systemic.

Local effects occur when visceral fat is deposited around your heart and blood vessels. This fat physically surrounds the heart and its blood vessels, and it interferes with the way the blood vessels behave by stopping them from relaxing fully. The fat also increases inflammation in the area around it, which further interferes with the normal function of your heart and blood vessels. Plus, this visceral fat can also get into the actual heart muscle cells themselves, with the result that your heart won't function as well as it should. If you're carrying extra weight, you really want a heart that's healthy, because it's going to have to work harder than the heart of a lighter person.

Systemic effects occur throughout the body. They result from fat accumulating in your liver, muscles and abdomen. So far, two key mechanisms have been identified. First, the presence of fat cells in these organs stops them from functioning the way they are supposed to. For example, your liver performs many vital functions, including removing waste products from your blood – it's

109

your very own in-house detox machine. When your liver has too much fat in it, it starts to malfunction and this can have wide-reaching effects. Second, the visceral fat itself can produce substances that have systemic effects. Some of these substances have been shown to be involved in the development of systemic inflammation and insulin resistance. All too often, the upshot is type 2 diabetes or metabolic syndrome.

So, why do we store visceral fat if it's so bad for us? The jury is still out on this, but it appears that our bodies do this as a last resort. The amount of subcutaneous fat your body can store depends on factors like your genes, age, gender, what you eat and whether or not you smoke, and there seems to be a limit to the amount that can be stored. Once that storage space is full, your body has to put any excess fat somewhere else, so it tucks it away in cells that aren't designed to store fat or puts it around the outside of organs – wherever it can find space. So if you have a lot of fat under your skin, there's a good chance that you've also got a lot of fat even deeper, slowly suffocating you from the inside out.

DID YOU KNOW?

The average age of a fat cell is 10 years.

MORE THAN YOU NEED?

Watch TV, read a magazine or surf the internet, and you can't help but notice all the talk about obesity. This isn't surprising, because the statistics are shocking. In many countries – including New Zealand, Australia, the UK and the US – around two-thirds of the population is classed as overweight or obese. That means that anyone who is underweight or within the 'approved' weight range is in a minority.

Of course, these figures are estimates. It's not like we have a

OECD AND OBESITY

A 2017 OECD report on obesity showed the extent of the problem in member countries. The top five countries for adult obesity were:

1. United States – 38.2%
2. Mexico – 32.4%
3. New Zealand – 30.7%
4. Hungary – 30%
5. Australia – 27.9%

'Weight Census' every four years, where someone comes around with a pair of scales and a tape measure! Yet, unbelievably, things might be even worse than those numbers indicate.

The usual way to measure whether or not someone is overweight is to use the BMI – the body mass index. To do this, you divide your weight (in kilograms) by the square of your height (in metres). So, for a person who was 1.83 metres tall and weighed 90 kg, the equation would be 90 divided by 3.35 (which is 1.83 x1.83) – which would give them a BMI of 26.8. This would put them in the overweight category (see the BMI panel overleaf).

Although BMI has been used for years, nowadays most people agree that it's not perfect. If you're very muscular, for example, you're quite likely to have a higher BMI just because muscle weighs more than fat. Many professional athletes – think rugby players, not marathon runners! – fall into the obese category simply because they have so much muscle.

Having extra weight as muscle isn't a health hazard – in fact, it's just the opposite. As mentioned earlier, muscle burns energy, helps protect your joints, ligaments and tendons – and, of course, helps you do any activity you want. What *is* a health hazard is having extra weight as fat – especially visceral fat.

However, measuring the amount of fat a body contains is notoriously difficult. If you have access to a fully equipped

BMI

The most widely used BMI groupings for adults are:
 # less than 18.5 = underweight
 # 18.5 to 24.9 = ideal weight
 # 25 to 29.9 = overweight
 # over 30 = obese

physiology lab that specialises in this sort of thing, you could have a DEXA scan, you could be weighed underwater, or you could sit in a BodPod. All of these will cost money, some more than others, and they're out of the question for most people, especially as you'd need to go back for more assessments if you wanted to see whether your body fat percentage had changed.

To monitor your body fat at home, you could invest in a set of bioelectrical impedance scales. These scales use a tiny electric current that runs through your body. The electricity travels at different rates through lean and fat tissue, and this is used to calculate body fat percentage. To get good readings – and good comparisons over time – you need to follow the instructions carefully.

You could also go old school, and use a set of body fat callipers to take measurements at various points on your body. You'd then put those into an online calculator that takes your weight, height, gender and age into account, and would get an estimate of your body fat that way. The challenge here is taking the measurements in the right places – and for some systems you need to have someone else take measurements unless you're very flexible and can measure skinfolds on your own back!

All of these approaches have their place, but they also have their limitations. None of them directly measures visceral fat – and this is the fat that most of us should be worried about.

Recently, some new measurements have been proposed – waist circumference, waist-to-hip ratio and waist-to-height ratio. These are all very easy to do and, importantly, they focus on the area of the body that expands as we accumulate visceral fat.

- # **Waist circumference:** The World Health Organization suggests that the risk of suffering from a weight-related metabolic disease is lower if your waist circumference is less than 94 cm for a man or less than 80 cm for a woman.
- # **Waist-to-hip ratio:** This has fallen out of favour recently, as it appears that it doesn't add much value. If you want to try it, divide your waist measurement by your hip measurement. For women, a ratio of 0.8 or below indicates low risk of metabolic health issues. For men, the target ratio is 0.95 or below.
- # **Waist-to-height ratio:** The newest kid on the block, this is another simple measurement that can be done at home. Measure your waist and your height (without shoes). If your waist is less than half your height, you're considered to be in the healthy category.

Unfortunately, not many people fall into the healthy category. A study from 2017 estimated that the vast majority of adults in New Zealand and Australia are 'overfat' (see the graphics overleaf). Overfat is not obese; it's not even overweight. People who are classed as overfat have excess body fat and, typically, it's visceral fat. Overfat matters because, as mentioned above, it's our visceral fat that leads to health problems like diabetes, cardiovascular issues, joint pain and a general lowering of quality of life.

A person can have a normal BMI and still be overfat, so what does overfat look like? Typically, it's the 'apple' body shape – skinny (or not) legs and arms, and a round, solid-looking middle. It's the body type often associated with men who have let the 'dad bod' get away on them. Since women are usually more pear-shaped, with more weight stored around their hips and thighs, when they get overfat the apple shape isn't so obvious. Ultimately, if your waist circumference is more than half your height, you're most likely overfat.

OVERFAT AND OVER HERE

A survey of the world's 30 most developed countries found that overfat is far more widespread than obesity. The winners (or maybe we should say losers!) in the overfat stakes were the USA, Iceland, New Zealand, the UK and Australia:

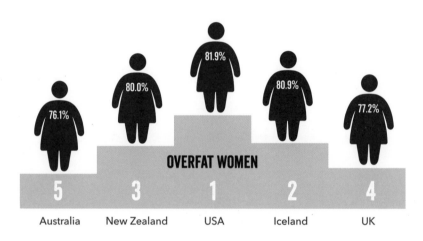

| 5 | 3 | 1 | 2 | 4 |
| Australia | New Zealand | USA | Iceland | UK |

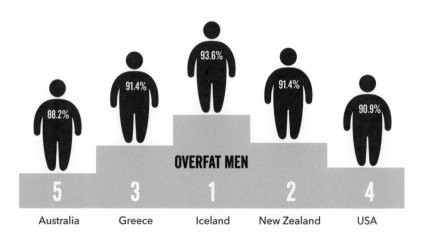

| 5 | 3 | 1 | 2 | 4 |
| Australia | Greece | Iceland | New Zealand | USA |

WHAT YOU CAN DO

Can you be fat and fit? Possibly. It depends which studies you look at, which criteria you use for assessment, and which populations you're studying.

If you're overfat, are you likely to get health benefits from losing a bit of that excess adipose tissue? Almost certainly. But if you go too far and become too lean, you'll also start to damage your health. There's a middle road where health and weight complement each other – and that's what we should aim for.

Of course, that middle road isn't a single number on the scales. Aiming to be exactly your target weight is almost always a recipe for disaster. Your bodyweight naturally fluctuates day to day – a large meal will drive it higher, a hot day when you sweat a lot will make it fall. For women in particular, hormonal activity will cause their bodyweight to move up and down. If you say 'I must be 62 kg or else', and then feel miserable because you've jumped on the scales and they say you're 62.5 kg, what does that do for your mental health? It's crazy – and it's no way to live.

It's much more realistic to aim to stay within a weight range that's good for you. That range might be as wide as 10 kg. For instance, you might think that in a perfect world you'd like to weigh 62 kg. But none of us is perfect, and we don't live in a perfect world either. So instead, set yourself a weight range that you're comfortable with – let's say a low of 62 kg and a high of 70 kg. Tell yourself that if you're within that range, you can be happy. But if you start drifting towards the top of the range, use that as a trigger to make small adjustments to your lifestyle so that you don't end up exceeding your upper limit.

What you'll probably find is that you'll tend to be at the lighter end of your range during summer, and at the heavier end during winter. This reflects our typical eating and activity patterns. In summer we're outdoors more and are more active, and our food tends to be lighter, especially if we live in a warmer area. In winter, we spend more time indoors, and have warming, comforting, filling food.

The most important thing to remember is that whether or not you can keep within your target weight range will mainly be influenced by what you eat – and how much you eat. Although popular websites, fitness gurus and reality-TV shows often promote exercise as being essential for weight loss, most studies show that *diet* is the main factor governing long-term weight loss. That said, crash diets and the like are *not* going to do your health any good. Yes, you might lose a bit of weight – and quite quickly – but it's not a sustainable way to live. Severe dieting is likely to lower your resting metabolic rate, which dictates the amount of energy you burn at rest. A lower resting metabolic rate means that your body requires fewer calories to run its basic systems. In time, this makes it easier for you to eat more calories than you need and to put on weight.

If you need more convincing that extreme dieting is not the way to manage your weight, look no further than the TV programme *The Biggest Loser*. A study of 14 successful competitors in this show found that they had lost an average of 58 kg over the 30-week programme – an astonishing achievement. However, over that same period their resting metabolic rates had dropped by an average of nearly 700 calories per day and – even worse – it was still that low six years later. As a result of that extreme weight loss attempt, these people now needed to eat, on average, 700 calories a day *fewer* just to maintain their weight. Not surprisingly, nearly all of them had regained at least some of the weight they'd lost – and some were actually heavier than before they'd appeared on the show.

A healthy daily diet with a focus on fresh food that's high in nutrients will be *so* much better for you in the long run. It's going to keep you healthy – it's going to actually *feed* your body, not starve it. It's going to allow you to build strong bones and powerful muscles, and that's going to help you use your body to live a great life.

#15 THE INVISIBLE INFLUENCERS

WHAT YOUR BODY DOES

Why do you get hungry? On one level the answer is simple – you haven't eaten enough! But how does your body know this? The answer to this is extremely complicated, and will probably only get more complicated as we do more research into it.

Pretty much everything your body does is regulated by hormones. These are signalling substances that get released by various tissues with the sole aim of causing an effect somewhere else in the body. Hormones make you go to sleep, make you wake up, regulate your sex drive and a host of other activities. Hunger is no different. Some hormones stimulate your appetite – perhaps the most widely known of these is ghrelin, which is mainly produced by your stomach. Other hormones suppress your appetite – the best known is probably leptin, which is produced by white fat cells (the ones that store excess energy as fat). Your brain also produces hormones that affect appetite.

All of these hormones work together in a complicated choreography to make you feel hungry, to switch other digestive hormones on or off, and to make you feel full – or, at least, not so hungry any more!

THE INS AND OUTS OF INSULIN

One of the substances affected by the hunger-hormone brigade is insulin. This hormone plays a critical role in helping the food that you eat actually get into your cells, where it can be used to produce energy, build new bits of your body or just get stored away for a hungry day.

Insulin is produced by the pancreas, and is released into your bloodstream even if you're not eating – although only in tiny amounts. Take in some food, however, and insulin swings into action. The main trigger for its sudden release is the presence of glucose in the blood, but it's also released in response to the presence of other substances: amino acids (which are what proteins are made of), fatty acids (which are produced when fat is broken down in the digestive tract) and ketones (which are produced when fat is burned in tissues).

Insulin is a bit like a doorman at a fancy hotel, or a bouncer at a nightclub. It lets glucose into muscle cells and fat cells, and at the same time it stops glucose from leaving the liver. A healthy liver stores glucose – in the form of glycogen – for use as a short-term energy source. Insulin also lets amino acids into cells, where they can be used to make proteins, and it also causes fat to be made in the liver, white fat cells and muscle tissue.

Insulin is a key player in health. If you become resistant to its effects, then you can no longer get glucose into your cells and you'll have diabetes. As a result, your cells will starve and your blood glucose levels will soar. Some of that blood glucose leaves the body in urine – in fact, one of the very early ways to diagnose diabetes was to taste the patient's urine to see whether it was sweet! If you have diabetes, your body makes more and more urine to try to flush out the excess glucose from your blood, so you get very thirsty. When your blood sugar levels stay high, they end up damaging your tissues and this eventually leads to the terrible complications of diabetes: blindness, circulation and nerve problems (which can lead to gangrene and amputation), strokes, kidney failure and heart attacks.

There are two main forms of diabetes. Type 1 is an auto-immune disease and is not associated with lifestyle choices. Type 2 is far more common and is on the rise all over the world. It's usually associated with insulin resistance, but not always – sometimes your body just doesn't produce enough insulin. Your genes play a role in determining whether or not you are at risk of developing diabetes – but lifestyle is even more important, and can override your genetic risk.

STRESSING OUT

If you thought that insulin was important for maintaining a healthy body, wait until you read about cortisol. This is produced by your adrenal glands, which sit on top of your kidneys. It's transported all around the body and has different effects on different cells.

The thing that cortisol is best known for is its role in stress. When you encounter a stress – like a huge credit card bill, working late *yet* again, or some idiot on the road nearly hitting you – cortisol leaps into action. One of the first things it does is make large amounts of glucose available to your body, so that you've got the energy you need to either fight or run away. To make sure that this glucose doesn't get put back into the cells, it reduces the activity of insulin. Also, to make sure that your muscles get the oxygen they might need, cortisol makes the arteries narrow so that the heart pumps faster, sending blood round the body more quickly.

Once the stress has subsided, cortisol levels fall and your body returns to normal. The problem for some people today is that stress hardly ever subsides. They go from a frantic morning trying to get out of the house, to sitting in crushing traffic congestion – or dealing with delayed trains and buses – to conflict in the workplace, to desktop dining, more conflict – or boredom – more traffic, and then maybe a nice family argument to finish it all off. No wonder we're stressed!

If this is your lifestyle, then your cortisol levels might be chronically elevated. And *that* will affect your health. Persistently high cortisol levels may increase your risk of developing type 2 diabetes for two reasons: (1) because they cause high blood glucose levels; and (2) because they effectively make your cells resistant to insulin. The fact that glucose can't get into some of your cells means that these cells are starved of energy, and that can trigger the release of hormones that increase your appetite – which makes you eat more. At the same time, cortisol increases your desire for high-calorie foods. Ever wonder why you get a craving for a chocolate bar or a doughnut when you've got a deadline looming and you're way behind schedule? That'll be your cortisol taking charge.

Just to make your life even more difficult, cortisol also helps move triglycerides out of storage in the liver and into visceral fat cells – the ones around your organs; you know: the ones you want to keep relatively empty. And just in case those fat cells get

YOUR BODY IS OUT TO GET YOU

Dieting increases your cortisol levels. Anyone who's ever been on a diet knows just how stressful it can be - restricting food intake is not fun. And it seems that the stress you feel in your mind is also felt in your body.

Scientists have known for a long time that when people fast or are starved, their cortisol levels increase. However, it has recently been shown that just going on a diet is enough to raise your cortisol. What's going on? No one knows for certain, but it could be that when you reduce your energy intake, your body produces more cortisol in an effort to release the energy stored in your body so that your cells have got enough fuel to function. The question is, does this elevated cortisol contribute to post-diet weight gain? The jury on this is still out for humans, but in rodents it does appear to play a role.

too full, cortisol also helps new fat cells develop!

Yet another function of cortisol is to reduce inflammation. If your lifestyle is causing your body to suffer from constant inflammation, then your cortisol levels will be chronically elevated. Triggers for this state include a poor diet, inadequate sleep and regular stress. Unless you make changes to your lifestyle, your body will end up fighting a losing battle trying to get this inflammation under control. The inflammation makes you more susceptible to a range of diseases and disorders, because (1) your immune system is compromised; and (2) the elevated cortisol levels make you eat and make you fat!

Cortisol has also been linked to a host of other health issues, including gastrointestinal problems, cardiovascular disease, fertility difficulties, insomnia, depression and dementia.

ELEVATING ENDORPHINS

Insulin and cortisol both play important roles in our health, but too much of these hormones can be detrimental to our long-term wellbeing. This doesn't seem to be the case with endorphins.

The term 'endorphin' covers a number of different compounds that are made by your body in one place and have effects in another place. These substances have an opiate-like quality – they help to reduce your perception of pain, and in doing so provide you with the perception of pleasure. Endorphins are most commonly associated with the 'runner's high' – the feeling of total relaxation and elation that some people get after they've tackled some sort of demanding physical exercise. That feeling is so pleasurable that some people choose to get it by other means – like opiate drugs. The active ingredient in opium binds to exactly the same receptors on your cells as your naturally produced endorphins do.

Taking opiates – or any illegal drug – is clearly not part of a healthy lifestyle. However, encouraging the release of your own natural endorphins *is*.

WHAT YOU CAN DO

You might not be able to see the hormones that run your body, but you *will* feel the effects if they get out of hand. Maintaining a healthy lifestyle will definitely help reduce your chances of having metabolic problems arising from hormonal imbalances.

TARGET THE TRIGGERS

The obvious hormone to target is insulin. This won't be news to you – the internet is saturated with talk about the effects of too much sugar in the diet. Table sugar, honey, maple syrup, agave syrup, coconut sugar, high-fructose corn syrup – it's pretty much all the same thing. If you want to eliminate it completely from your diet, then feel free – but make sure you're going to enjoy that lifestyle, or you won't be able to sustain it.

If you like sweet foods, try working out which ones you really want to keep in your life – and ditch the rest. If, for example, you really like home-made cake but find shop-bought ones a bit *meh*, consider making a pact with yourself to only eat home-made cake. That way, if you're at work or a birthday party and someone brings some home-baking, you can have a bit without beating yourself up. The same principle applies if your thing is chocolate, or ice cream, or any other sweet treat. If you really like dark chocolate, consider giving up eating milk chocolate and white chocolate. If you really like ice cream, is there a single flavour or type you could restrict yourself to? Another way to tackle this is to allow yourself to eat anything – but only on the weekends.

Whichever way you choose to moderate the amount of sugar in your diet, the only thing that matters is that *it works for you*. You know what you like and what you're prepared to give up – so don't let someone else tell you what to do. Instead, build a healthy approach to sugar on your own terms.

Of course, it's not just cakes and chocolate that trigger an insulin response. Fizzy drinks are a shocker for this, as are pastries, bread, pasta, rice and even potatoes. Managing your consumption of these types of food will help to keep your insulin levels under control.

Maintaining a healthy, balanced lifestyle will help keep other hormones in check, too – including cortisol. The key here is to minimise the amount of stress that's in your life each day. So, if you find yourself getting tense because you've missed a workout or eaten one too many biscuits, see whether you can't cut yourself some slack. Everyone skips the odd workout or indulges occasionally. Just accept that it's happened, and resolve to make tomorrow a better day.

TRACK YOUR TRENDS

If you're really keen to take control of your health, consider getting your doctor to do annual health checks. Ask your GP to do the obvious things like weight, blood pressure, skin check, etc., but also ask for a full blood screen. You – and your doctor – are likely to be interested in a number of different factors:

Your iron status – to check for anaemia (frequently caused by a lack of iron) or a condition where the body stores too much iron (haemochromatosis).

- \# Vitamin B_{12} and folic acid levels – low levels can lead to anaemia; low folic acid is also a risk factor for women who want to have children, as it increases the risk of neural tube defects in the developing foetus.
- \# Liver function tests – liver disorders can easily go unnoticed until they reach an advanced stage.
- \# Kidney function tests – especially if there is a family history of problems.
- \# Gender-specific tests – e.g. PSA for men, to check for prostate cancer.
- \# Cholesterol levels – to help assess your risk of cardiovascular disease.
- \# HbA1c test – to check your average blood sugar levels over the previous six weeks.

If your GP doesn't routinely do this type of assessment, you might find them asking why you've made this request. There are two good reasons you can discuss:

1. Getting these tests done every year means that if any test result starts to drift away from the normal range, it might just give you – and your doctor – enough advance warning so that you can catch and correct a disorder before it gets too serious.
2. You've got a chance to use the information you receive to alter your lifestyle so that you're adopting healthier behaviours.

For example, say that your HbA1c level was up towards the top of the acceptable range. If you currently take two sugars in your tea and have six cups a day, and have biscuits with two of those, plus you have a diet that's pretty high in white bread and pasta and potatoes, then you can choose to make some changes and see if these help to bring your HbA1c level down. You might simply halve the amount of sugar in your tea and halve the amount of carbohydrate in your meals. That reduction could be all that's needed – and even if it only stabilises your blood sugar levels, that's still better than having them creep gradually up and up until you're diabetic.

It's also important to remember that there is no one magic number for any of these tests. There's usually a range that is deemed 'acceptable'. For example, in a person without diabetes, an HbA1c of less than 40 mmol/mol is ideal, but if you have diabetes then slightly higher levels are considered normal.

Getting blood tests done can be scary, so this approach might not be right for you. Also, if you know that you won't take any action based on the outcome of the tests, then you're probably better off not taking them in the first place. You need to be prepared for the possibility of unwelcome news – whatever that might be. These are all things that you should discuss with your GP.

SLEEP TIGHT

Sleep's an overlooked part of health, but it is absolutely essential. When you're asleep, your body repairs the damage that's been done to its cells during the day. If you don't get enough sleep, it's not just your cells that suffer. Insufficient sleep has been shown to result in an increase in cortisol levels. Normally, cortisol falls in the evening before you go to sleep; but if you're not getting enough sleep, it doesn't fall as quickly, which is thought to increase your risk of insulin resistance, which in turn puts you at greater risk of developing type 2 diabetes. The release of growth hormone is also altered, and this is likely to have an adverse effect on glucose tolerance, further increasing your risk of metabolic illness.

Not only that, but a lack of sleep also makes you more hungry – and again, it's driven by changes in hormone levels. When you're sleep-deprived, your levels of leptin fall and those of ghrelin rise. Leptin tells your brain that you're not hungry – so if levels are low, your brain thinks that your body needs food. Ghrelin tells your brain that you *are* hungry – so if levels rise, your brain thinks that your body needs food. Putting this together, if you're sleep-deprived then you have *two* hormone systems telling your brain that you need doughnuts and pastries – and that you need them *now!* (Studies have shown that sleep-deprived people crave carbohydrate-rich food, rather than bacon and eggs.) And that extra food isn't just needed because you're awake for longer and are therefore burning more energy. The additional calorie intake will exceed what you'd burn during that time, meaning that you're quite likely to gain weight.

A lot of people don't get enough sleep. A study in 2013 found that 1 in 3 of the people who were surveyed got less than 8 hours sleep a night, and 60% of those questioned said they would like more sleep.

Eight hours of sleep is generally recommended, but for many people 9 hours might be more appropriate. So, how do you achieve this?

1. The first step is to make it a priority! How many times do you think you should go to bed but instead choose to watch another hour of TV? Make it a priority to get 9 hours of sleep a night, and that way you should stand a good chance of getting at least 8.

2. Establish a routine, so that at a set time – say 9 pm – you start getting ready to go to bed. Then, over the next hour, de-power. Do something relaxing – meditate, take a bath or shower, do some deep breathing, read a book, do your ironing, listen to music, do some foam rolling.

3. When you go to bed, make sure that the room is dark. Electric lights and iPad screens weren't around when we evolved. Use a dimmer on your light if you have one, and don't pick up your phone or tablet.

4. Try to have your bedroom at a comfortable temperature – if it's too hot or too cold, you won't sleep well. Somewhere between 17 and 19 °C is ideal. If it's too cold, have a warm shower or bath, or wear a pair of cosy socks to bed. If it's too hot, get the room as cool as possible well before you go to bed, and keep your bedding to a minimum.

5. Quiet also helps. If you live in a noisy area – say you're on a busy street or you have the neighbours from hell – then invest in a good pair of earplugs.

There are also a couple of food tricks that can help you get a good night's sleep. Tart cherry juice has been shown to increase levels of melatonin, a hormone that promotes sleep, and people taking this juice sleep longer. Eating two kiwifruit an hour before going to bed has been shown to reduce the amount of time it takes to fall asleep, and to increase the length of time you actually sleep.

Of course, if you have a coffee just before your kiwifruit, you'll probably completely negate any benefits. For most people, coffee and other caffeinated drinks are best avoided after mid-afternoon. It's important to stay hydrated, though, as this will also affect the quality of your sleep – so be sure to drink water and low-caffeine, sugar-free drinks instead.

Finally, if you find that you just haven't had enough sleep and are struggling to make it through the day, see whether you can take a power nap. Just 15–20 minutes is all that's needed – any longer, and you'll make it more difficult to sleep that night. Set a timer, lie down, shut your eyes and relax. Even if you don't actually fall asleep, you'll still get a benefit from doing this.

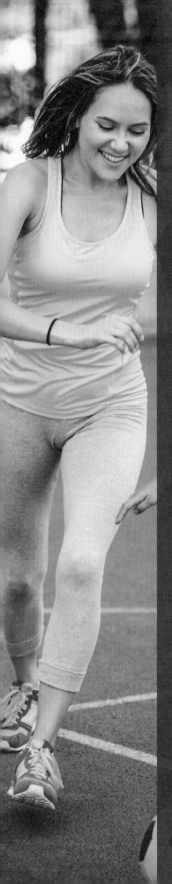

ANYONE CAN DO THIS

Louise, 42

With three active boys at home and a busy full-time job that sees me away from home a lot, I need to be fit and healthy just to cope! And luckily for me, I've always been fit and active. But despite that, I felt like I was stuck. I wanted to see if I could get more out of myself – without compromising on my work or family life – so I signed up for Nic's programme, which was being offered through work.

My idea of a healthy person is someone who has a strong body and eats clean, raw nutrition to fuel that body – it's something that we strive for as a family, eating real food and doing lots of different outdoor activities together. I was interested to see whether Nic had anything more to offer us. My personal goals were to get leaner and faster – and I'm happy to say that I achieved both of these. I'm now leaner than I have ever been in my life, and my running is faster and easier than ever before.

There were two ideas that Nic proposed that helped make that difference. One was to start the day by drinking a minimum of 500 ml of water – I just sip away while I'm pottering around in the kitchen getting the breakfasts and lunchboxes ready. It's so easy and so simple. The other is his 10-minute kickers: if I don't have time for anything else, I can always find time for these. There's no way I'm trying his cold showers, though!

If someone was thinking of following Nic's advice, I'd say go for it. I've got an incredibly hectic schedule, with long-haul flights, sleep deprivation and long periods away from home, and if I can do it with all of those demands on my time, then anyone can.

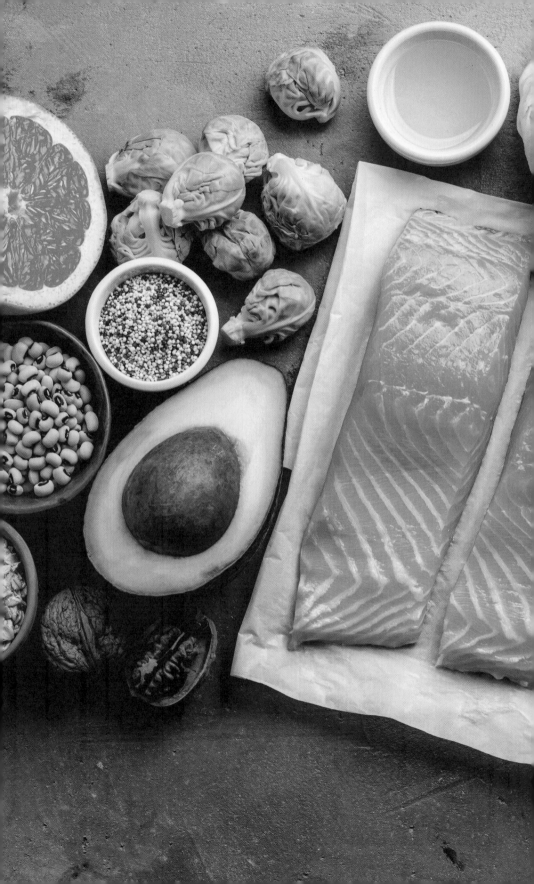

PART
FOUR

—

INSIDE
YOUR
GUT

Maybe you didn't take any science subjects at school. Maybe you've become confused by all the information that's available today. Maybe you've never given it a second thought. Whatever your 'maybe', there's a strong chance that you're not 100% certain about what macronutrients, micronutrients and phytonutrients are — or what they do or why they are important. Without this knowledge, it's really difficult to appreciate the health impacts of the food you put into your body. Instead, you'll focus on the immediate reward — the feeling of contentment and satisfaction that comes from a full stomach, the delicious taste of something high in fat, sugar or salt, or the mood-altering effect of a glass of wine or a cup of coffee. Once you understand the fundamentals of nutrition, you're in a far better position to make informed choices about your food. You can deliberately opt for foods that you know are beneficial for your health, or you can eat or drink something in full knowledge that it's not the optimum choice, and elect to compensate for that with your other food choices that day.

#16
CARBOHYDRATES – SIMPLE AND COMPLEX

Carbohydrates are found in most foodstuffs. Bread, potatoes, kiwifruit and steak all contain some form of carbohydrate. Chemically, carbohydrates consist of three elements - carbon, hydrogen and oxygen. These combine together in rings to form a range of different sugars, or saccharides as scientists call them.

SIMPLE CARBS

Monosaccharides are the simplest of the sugars. As the 'mono' part of their name suggests, they contain just one carbohydrate ring. Common monosaccharides in the human diet include glucose (used by the body to produce energy), fructose (found in fruit) and galactose (found in milk). Honey contains a range of different sugars, mainly fructose and glucose. Agave syrup is mostly fructose.

Disaccharides together are formed when two monosaccharides join together. Sucrose - or table sugar - is a disaccharide made up of one ring of fructose and one ring of glucose. Sucrose is produced naturally by plants. Most of our sugar comes from either sugar beet or sugar cane. Coconut sugar, one of the internet sensations of 2017, also contains sucrose - about 80%.

COMPLEX CARBS

Anything more complex than a disaccharide is called a **polysaccharide** ('poly' means many). There are three main groups of polysaccharides found in foods:

1. **Starches:** Energy-storage compounds found in a wide range of foods, including vegetables, grains and legumes. Starches can be digested by humans.

2. **Cellulose:** Along with a range of other materials, comprises the structural material of plants. Cellulose cannot be digested by humans.

3. **Glycogen:** This polysaccharide is found in the muscles and liver of animals. It is readily digested by humans. Glycogen stored in your own body is broken down and used for energy when other sources of energy are in short supply.

CARBS AND ENERGY

Inside your body, glucose is used to produce energy. A series of biochemical reactions chops the glucose ring into two straight molecules called pyruvate. At the same time, this process produces two molecules of ATP, which is the compound that provides the energy for metabolic reactions. If oxygen is available, the pyruvate is further broken down to produce water and carbon dioxide, along with a lot more ATP. If there's not enough oxygen, the pyruvate is converted to lactate – this is the cause of the lactic acid burn you can experience during high-intensity exercise.

If there's more glucose available than is immediately required for energy, that glucose is converted to glycogen. This happens in the liver. Glycogen is used as a short-term storage system. When you have breakfast, your body uses some of that food energy right away and pops the excess into glycogen storage. Then, as you require energy during the day, that glycogen is released into the bloodstream and converted back to glucose to fuel your cells.

If you eat a diet that's high in simple sugars – disaccharides and monosaccharides – your body doesn't have to work very hard to use that energy. It's available pretty much instantly. It doesn't take much effort for your body to chop disaccharides into two monosaccharides and then convert these into glucose.

When you eat starches, the process is a bit slower. How much slower depends very much on the type of starch. Some can be broken into glucose quite rapidly, while others take much longer. The digestion of starches begins in the mouth, where an enzyme (alpha-amylase) breaks some of the more accessible bonds. This continues in the stomach until the enzyme is inactivated by the acidic environment. When the food moves into the small intestine it gets another dose of alpha-amylase, this time from the pancreas. This breaks the starch into smaller pieces, known as oligosaccharides. Other enzymes then produce disaccharides, which are eventually cut into monosaccharides. All this happens in the small intestine, and the monosaccharides are absorbed from there into the bloodstream. From there, they enter the energy-producing, glucose-burning system described above.

The speed at which a polysaccharide is broken down to monosaccharides depends in part on its structure and in part on what else is eaten with it. Starches contain two structures – amylose and amylopectin. Both are made up of thousands of glucose units, but amylose is relatively short and unbranched (like a sapling), while amylopectin is up to 100,000 times larger and extensively branched (like a huge old oak tree). The structure affects how easily and how quickly they can be digested.

Chewing food thoroughly helps to break it down into smaller pieces so that digestion can occur more quickly. However, eating carbohydrate together with fibre, fat and/or protein slows the digestive process, resulting in lower blood concentrations of glucose, insulin and cholesterol after a meal.

FIBRE FACTS

If you eat a healthy diet, you probably get enough fibre. But most of us don't. Fibre is the indigestible portion of food – it's found in all sorts of plant material, from leafy greens to whole grains to beans and even fruits. There are two types of fibre – soluble and insoluble.

WHAT IS RESISTANT STARCH?

Most starch is easily digested by the human body, but resistant starch isn't – instead, it passes right through us, pretty much untouched. There are several different types of resistant starch. One type resists digestion because it's physically hard to get to – it's incorporated into the fibrous cell walls of grains, seeds and legumes. Another type is resistant because of its chemical form – it's found in unripe foods like raw potatoes and green bananas.

Very recently, attention has been focused on a third type, which develops when some starchy foods are cooked and then cooled. During the cooling process, the amylose chains in the starch start to take on a much more orderly structure, so they become more like a crystal. When you eat a food that's gone through this process, less of the amylose chains is exposed to the alpha-amylase enzymes in your digestive tract, so the starch is more resistant to digestion.

Resistant starch might be unavailable to us, but it is an excellent food source for the micro-organisms that live in our lower digestive tract. Bacteria in the large intestine (colon) digest the resistant starch and produce short-chain fatty acids. These include butyrate, which is used as fuel by the cells that line the colon. Adequate levels of butyrate in the large intestine may help to maintain gut health. Butyrate has also been shown to help repair damaged DNA, which may in turn help reduce the chance of you developing colon cancer.

When consumed in the form of whole plant foods (unprocessed grains, legumes and starchy vegetables), resistant starch is believed to have several health benefits, including reducing inflammation, improving digestion, improving blood cholesterol and fat levels, and helping us feel fuller for longer. Not bad for something that we can't digest!

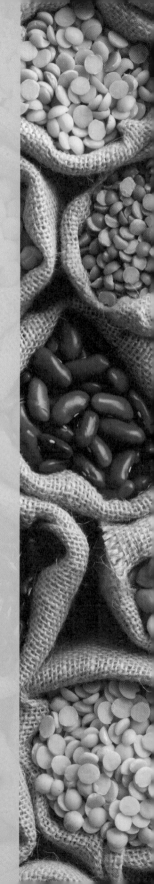

Soluble fibre gets its name because it can dissolve in water. Foods such as oats, nuts, pulses and fruits are, typically, good sources of soluble fibre. When we eat foods containing soluble fibre, the fibre absorbs water and forms a gel, which passes through our small intestine relatively untouched. Once in the large intestine, the soluble fibre becomes food for the bacteria that live there. Compounds that do this are called prebiotics, and they occur naturally in food – they don't need to be taken as pills or specialised, expensive drinks.

Insoluble fibre doesn't dissolve in water. This is the 'roughage' in our diet. It comes from the structural parts of plants – the cell walls that need to be tough and rigid so that the plant doesn't just flop over and lie on the ground. This fibre remains relatively untouched all the way through our digestive system. It still has an important role, however – it keeps things moving through your digestive system so that you don't get constipation!

In New Zealand and Australia, the recommended dietary intake of fibre is 25 g/day for women and 30 g/day for men. A 2011 study in New Zealand showed that average intakes are significantly lower than this – just 17.5 g/day for women and 22.1 g/day for men. Studies in similarly developed countries have shown the same sort of pattern. It seems pretty clear that we are all falling short of our fibre intake targets!

CARBOHYDRATES IN THE CUPBOARD (AND OTHER PLACES)

Here's a breakdown of some of the carbohydrates you're likely to find in a typical Western diet, along with some of their good and bad points.

CARBOHYDRATE SOURCE	FEATURES
Bread (white, brown, wholemeal, sourdough, garlic, etc.)	All bread is made from milled grains, which means it will be digested quickly. A wholemeal or sourdough bread offers a small nutritional advantage over a white supermarket-style loaf, but both mainly provide calories.
Pasta (white, wholemeal)	All pasta is made from milled grains, which means it will be digested quickly. Cooking pasta *al dente* slows the rate at which it is digested, but it still remains mainly a source of calories.
Rice (white, brown, Arborio, red, black, etc.)	Unmilled varieties contain resistant starch and fibre, but fibre is missing from all white varieties (basmati, jasmine, Arborio, Carnaroli, etc.). Rice mainly provides calories.
Potatoes, kumara, taro	These contain resistant starch and fibre, but their value depends on how they are prepared. Baking with the skin on retains most of the nutritional value of these vegetables.
Commercial breakfast cereals	These are mostly made from processed or milled grains, and usually contain added sugar (sometimes in multiple forms). They may be fortified with minerals. Cereals that are highly processed (i.e. they don't look like the raw ingredients) will be digested quickly.
Barley, oats and other whole grains	In their whole, uncooked form, these contain high amounts of fibre, along with complex carbohydrate. Processing (e.g. rolling of oats, pearling of barley) speeds up the rate at which they will be digested.
Fruits	Contain fibre and sugars, along with minerals, vitamins and sometimes phytonutrients.
Fizzy drinks	Contain sugar! Digested rapidly, causing a blood glucose and insulin spike.
Fruit juices	Contain sugar! Some may contain a small amount of fibre, minerals and vitamins.

Milk and milk drinks	Contain sugar in the form of lactose, along with minerals and vitamins.
Sugar (white, brown, caster, icing, raw, coconut, etc.)	These are just sugar! Digested rapidly, causing a blood glucose and insulin spike.
Jam, honey and syrups (golden syrup, rice syrup, agave, maple syrup, etc.)	Contain a lot of sugar! Digested rapidly, causing a blood glucose and insulin spike.
Cake, biscuits, sweets	Contain sugar and easily digested starches, since they are made from milled grains.
Beans and lentils	Contain resistant starch and fibre. They are also high in protein and provide vitamins, minerals and phytonutrients.
Pies and pastries	Made from milled grains, so will be digested rapidly although the rate may be slowed by the high fat content.
Sweetcorn	Contains resistant starch and fibre, along with digestible starch, vitamins, minerals and phytonutrients.
Quinoa	Contains relatively high amounts of fibre, along with protein, minerals and phytonutrients.

DIETITIAN OR NUTRITIONIST?

A dietitian is specifically trained in human nutrition - which includes postgraduate qualifications - and has to be registered and hold a practising certificate.
Anyone can call themselves a nutritionist, although some do have qualifications and are registered with their industry body.
Be sure to check so that you *know* you are getting informed advice, rather than just someone's opinion!

THE WORLD IS OUT TO GET YOU

Most of us do most of our food shopping in a supermarket – it's so easy, especially when you're busy. So we dash in, maybe we grab some carrots, some potatoes and a bag of apples, then a bottle of wine (or two!), and then we get to the grocery part of the store – and here we are assailed by advertising. The food packaging in those aisles is blinged to the max. Bright colours, bold type, seductive design – marketing professionals know exactly what will catch your eye and entice you to hand over your money. The next thing you know, you've got two boxes of unicorn pizza, four tins of rainbow spaghetti and a six-pack of super-berry smoothie satisfaction in your trolley.

How do you avoid this happening time and time again? There are plenty of strategies, but the best way is to avoid these aisles altogether, unless they contain items that are on your shopping list. In other words shop the perimeter. The perimeter typically has all the power points. The real, whole, colourful foods that need chilling – not white, dull, energy-laden, chemically filled food with a shelf life of twelve months.

Food marketing might be a relatively new activity, but it's incredibly powerful and effective. Two of the strategies that marketers use to entice you to buy their products are to focus on what the product doesn't have in it, and to hype up an ingredient that the product does contain. Here are some examples:

- # '99% sugar-free beer'.
- # 'Fat-free marshmallows'.
- # 'No artificial colours, flavours or preservatives'.
- # 'Oven-baked, not fried'.
- # '50% less added sugar'.
- # 'Made with real fruit'.
- # 'Fortified with vitamins and minerals'.

So, what's the matter with these claims? They're all true, but they're also a bit misleading:

- # Beer has very little sugar in it anyway – less than 1g per 500 ml – so the claim is meaningless. But it makes you think that this product is better for you than other beers that don't say the same thing.

Similarly, marshmallows never contain fat – they're made with sugar, gelatine, water and flavouring.

A product may well have no 'artificial' ingredients, but that doesn't mean it's free from things that can damage your health. Sugar is a natural food, but no one buys a bag of it because it's free of artificial colour, flavour or preservatives.

Advice to reduce our fat intake has led to snack foods that are 'oven-baked, not fried'. But these products are still usually made from hyper-processed grains of some sort, glued together in a shape that's designed to deliver visual, taste and crunch appeal. Just because they haven't seen the inside of a deep-fryer, that doesn't make them much healthier for us.

Products are often reformulated in response to current health concerns. For a while, it was all 'low-fat' or 'lower fat'. Now, it's all 'sugar-free', 'low in sugar' or 'reduced sugar'. A food that's advertising itself as having 50% less added sugar might still contain much more sugar in than you'd expect – it all depends on the starting point.

The 'Made with real fruit' statement can be found on a lot of products, from yoghurt to sweets to muesli bars and more. You never see it written on real fruit, though! The question to ask is how much real fruit there is in the product. You'll often find that it's a tiny amount – certainly not enough to offer any real nutritional benefit.

And as for foods that are 'Fortified with vitamins and minerals', ask yourself how nutritionally poor are these foods that they need to be fortified in this way?

Marketers want you to think that their products are the best, and that they're better for you than other products. If you can learn how to read labels, you'll be able to determine whether these products actually deliver what you're after from your food.

#17 THE PROTEIN STORY

Proteins are found in many foods. Some are obvious - red meat, fish, chicken; while some are less obvious - vegetables, grains, legumes. The main distinguishing feature of proteins is that they contain nitrogen. This nitrogen is a key component of the amino acids that combine to form the vast number of different proteins that exist.

When we eat foods that contain protein, enzymes in our digestive system break it down into its amino acid components (and some slightly larger fragments called peptides). This process starts in the stomach and continues in the small intestine, where the amino acids are absorbed into the bloodstream. Your body then uses these amino acids to build new tissue and repair damaged cells.

Unlike the carbohydrate digestion process, which is a bit wasteful, protein digestion is very efficient. In adults, about 98% of the protein that is eaten is absorbed by the body.

WHAT'S ESSENTIAL

Some of the amino acids your body needs can be manufactured by your body from the components that come in the food you eat. However, there are nine amino acids that your body can't make, so you need to eat foods containing these. At one time people believed that foods had to be combined to provide a complete balance of proteins at each meal, but that idea has long since been discarded. As long as your daily diet contains a variety of foodstuffs, it's likely to deliver all the amino acids you require.

How much protein do you need? Well, if you're not particularly physically active, you only need a mere 0.8 g protein per kg of bodyweight per day. For a 70 kg woman, that's 56 g per day; for a 100 kg man, that's 80 g per day. If you're doing a

HOW DO TAKEAWAYS STACK UP?

Many of us like a takeaway now and then – so what do they look like from a protein perspective?

A Big Mac will give you 26.7 g of protein – but it will also supply over 500 calories (and that's without any fries or a drink).

An individual mince pie will give you 13.3 g of protein – and around 460 calories (without any tomato sauce).

One deep-fried piece of fish will give you 22 g of protein – and about 440 calories (before you add chips, sauce and a pineapple fritter).

One slice of meat-lover's pizza will give you around 15 g of protein – and about 240 calories (but who can stop at one slice?)

lot of physical activity and trying to build up muscle mass, then you can double that allowance – hence the attraction of egg white omelettes and protein shakes for bodybuilders. A protein intake over 2 g protein per kg bodyweight per day would be regarded as high.

In developed countries a lack of protein is rarely an issue, except for some groups – older people tend to eat less and may not get enough protein, and people suffering from eating disorders and some medical conditions can also struggle to meet their protein needs. Mostly, though, we eat more protein than we require. A recent survey in New Zealand found the average intake to be 102 g/day for men and 71 g/day for women, with only 2% of the population not getting enough protein. These levels are enough to fuel a 127 kg man and an 89 kg woman, assuming that they both have office jobs, commute by car and do mainly sofa-based leisure activities. In Europe and the United

States, people typically eat one-and-a-half to two times as much protein as they need.

The arrival of the Atkins diet, the Paleo diet and similar approaches to food have really shone the spotlight on protein in recent times. With many of these regimes, it would be quite easy to eat significant quantities of protein. And not only does this get a bit expensive, but consuming excess protein over a long time can result in health problems. Too much for too long can cause digestive problems, may exacerbate kidney problems and could also affect the health of your blood vessels. And of course, if you're not using the energy that you consume in protein form, then you're going to gain weight.

PROTEINS IN THE PANTRY (AND OTHER PLACES)

Here's a breakdown of some of the protein food sources you're likely to find in a typical Western diet, along with some of their good and bad points.

PROTEIN SOURCE	FEATURES
Red meat	Contains a large amount of protein (a 150 g piece of steak provides about 40 g of protein), and includes essential amino acids. But it also adds saturated fat to the diet.
White meat	White meats like chicken are excellent sources of protein, with 100 g of meat providing around 30 g of protein.
Fish (white and oily)	All fish are a good source of protein. Oily fish also supplies omega-3 oils. A 150 g serving of salmon provides about 34 g of protein.
Dairy (cheese, yoghurt, milk)	A standard serving of cheddar (25 g) contains about 6 g of protein; a cup of milk contains 8.5 g; a 150 g serving of Greek yoghurt contains 7.5 g of protein.
Eggs	A plain two-egg omelette will give you 13 g of protein.
Legumes	Beans and lentils are a good source of protein, with 1 cup providing about 18 g of protein and 15 g of fibre.

Tofu and tempeh	Tofu is about 8% protein, while tempeh is nearer to 20%.
Nuts	All nuts are good protein sources, either whole or turned into butters. A tablespoon of peanut butter provides just under 4 g of protein.
Seeds	Seeds are high in protein, minerals and vitamins. Sunflower seeds are about 23% protein; pumpkin seeds are about 25%. Uncooked quinoa is 16% protein.
Vegetables	The protein content of vegetables varies: 1 cup of cooked broccoli provides about 6 g of protein, 1 cup of cooked carrots only about 1 g. A cup of sweetcorn provides about 5 g of protein, and a cup of green peas 9 g.
Grains	Whole grains provide more protein than processed grains.
Baked goods	Bread is the main source of protein in many people's diets, which reflects how often it is eaten. A slice of wholegrain bread contains about 4 g of protein.

#18 WHAT'S UP WITH FATS

If there's a macronutrient that's gone from hero to zero and back to hero again, then it's got to be fat. Before we all started fretting over what we ate, fat was a big part of the menu for many families. Butter was slathered on bread, roast potatoes were crisped up in lard, we had full-fat milk in tea and whipped cream on a pavlova. Fat was an integral part of everyday meals.

Then, in the 1970s, came the suggestion that fat intake was linked to heart disease. All those flavour-laden, fat-adorned items started disappearing from the table. Butter was replaced with margarine, 'skinny' and 'lite' versions of recipes started to appear in cookbooks, and low-fat dairy products filled the supermarket chillers.

However, as further scientific research was done, it became apparent that fat might not be quite so bad after all. Suddenly there was a division between 'good' fats and 'bad' fats – the latter being fats of animal origin, like butter and cheese and pork crackling. Olive oil – the poster child for good fats – entered our kitchens in full force, and it was accompanied by a host of other oils – canola, sunflower and the rather vague 'vegetable oil'.

The more the effects of fat on human health were investigated, the more complex the picture became, and so it was hardly surprising that diets promoting fat intake started to appear. From the Atkins diet (where you were allowed cream in your coffee but not milk), to the Paleo diet (which can end up as high-fat, depending on what you eat), to the low-carb, high-fat (LCHF) diet that was developed in Sweden to treat obesity-related diabetes, there are now many variations on the theme. If you choose to follow one of these, it's worth being aware of the different types of fat that you can eat, and what effects they might have on your health.

THE STRUCTURE OF FAT

The majority of fats occur as triglycerides – they have a 'spine' that's made of glycerol, with three fatty acids attached to it. These fatty acids can be different lengths, depending on how many carbon atoms they contain. For example, short-chain fatty acids have five or fewer carbons; butyrate (see page 134) is an example of a short-chain fatty acid (SCFA). Most of the fatty acids we consume are either medium (MCFA)- or long-chain (CLCFA) ones.

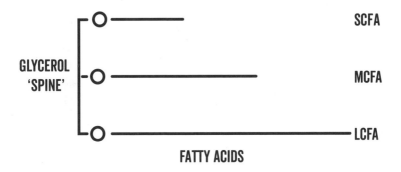

A carbon atom can form up to four bonds with itself (or other atoms). When all the bonds between the carbon atoms are single, then the fatty acid is said to be **saturated**. In other words, no more atoms can be added to the carbons in the chain. If one of those carbon atoms is connected to another with a double bond, then the fatty acid is called **monounsaturated**. If there is more than one double bond between the carbon atoms in the fatty acid, it's called **polyunsaturated**.

SATURATED

$$H-\overset{\overset{\displaystyle H}{|}}{\underset{\underset{\displaystyle H}{|}}{C}}-\overset{\overset{\displaystyle H}{|}}{\underset{\underset{\displaystyle H}{|}}{C}}-\overset{\overset{\displaystyle H}{|}}{\underset{\underset{\displaystyle H}{|}}{C}}-\overset{\overset{\displaystyle H}{|}}{\underset{\underset{\displaystyle H}{|}}{C}}-C\overset{\displaystyle O}{\underset{\displaystyle OH}{}}$$

MONOUNSATURATED

$$H-\overset{\overset{\displaystyle H}{|}}{\underset{\underset{\displaystyle H}{|}}{C}}-\overset{\overset{\displaystyle H}{|}}{\underset{\underset{\displaystyle H}{|}}{C}}-\overset{}{\underset{\underset{\displaystyle H}{|}}{C}}=\overset{}{\underset{\underset{\displaystyle H}{|}}{C}}-C\overset{\displaystyle O}{\underset{\displaystyle OH}{}}$$

POLYUNSATURATED

$$H-\overset{\overset{\displaystyle H}{|}}{\underset{\underset{\displaystyle H}{|}}{C}}-\overset{}{\underset{\underset{\displaystyle H}{|}}{C}}=\overset{}{\underset{}{C}}=\overset{}{\underset{\underset{\displaystyle H}{|}}{C}}-C\overset{\displaystyle O}{\underset{\displaystyle OH}{}}$$

There is one more structural aspect about unsaturated fatty acids that we need to understand, and that's the orientation of the hydrogen atoms. Single bonds will rotate, but double bonds are rigid. This means that the positions of hydrogen atoms at each end of a double bond are fixed. In most naturally occurring unsaturated fatty acids, the hydrogen atoms sit on the same side of the double bond. This is known as a 'cis' form. If the hydrogen atoms are on opposite sides, then the fatty acid changes shape and is called 'trans'. Trans fats were quite common in industrially produced oils until it was realised how damaging they are for human health.

CIS

$$H-\overset{\overset{\displaystyle H}{|}}{\underset{\underset{\displaystyle H}{|}}{C}}-\overset{\overset{\displaystyle H}{|}}{\underset{\underset{\displaystyle H}{|}}{C}}-\overset{\overset{\displaystyle H}{|}}{\underset{}{C}}=\overset{\overset{\displaystyle H}{|}}{\underset{}{C}}-C\overset{\displaystyle O}{\underset{\displaystyle OH}{}}$$

TRANS

$$H-\overset{\overset{\displaystyle H}{|}}{\underset{\underset{\displaystyle H}{|}}{C}}-\overset{\overset{\displaystyle H}{|}}{\underset{\underset{\displaystyle H}{|}}{C}}-\overset{\overset{\displaystyle H}{|}}{\underset{}{C}}=\overset{}{\underset{\underset{\displaystyle H}{|}}{C}}-C\overset{\displaystyle O}{\underset{\displaystyle OH}{}}$$

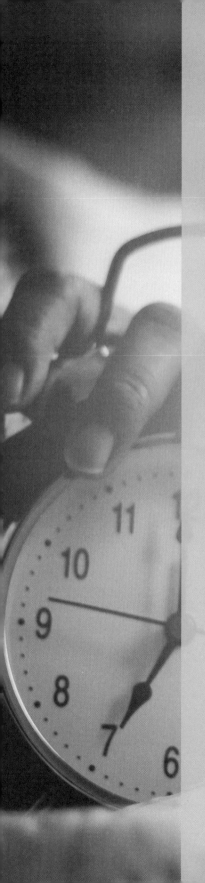

SLEEP SMART

Researchers have shown that eating fish improves sleep and makes you smarter! OK, so the work was done with children, but the benefits could still apply to adults. The researchers looked at the relationship between the frequency of eating fish, the duration and quality of sleep, and the IQ of the children. They found that including just one fish-based meal a week in the children's diet was associated with better sleep quality, and that children who ate this way scored an average of 4.8 points higher on an IQ test than children who didn't eat fish at all.

SFAS, MUFAS, PUFAS, AND MORE

Saturated fatty acids (SFAs) in the human diet mainly come from animal sources. Visible fat on meat, marbled fat in meat, the fat under the skin of a chicken, the fat in dairy products – this is all largely saturated fat. If you eat pastries, cakes, biscuits or any type of baked goods, you'll probably get saturated fat that way, too. Saturated fat makes great pastry!

It's long been thought that saturated fat is an influential factor in increasing the risk of cardiovascular disease. However, simply removing saturated fat from your diet may not be enough. Studies show that replacing saturated fat with carbohydrate doesn't produce the health benefits we'd expect. In fact, replacing saturated fat with digestible carbohydrate can result in blood markers indicating changes that are less favourable for cardiovascular health.

Monounsaturated fatty acids (MUFAs) occur in relatively high amounts in a relatively few vegetable sources. Olives and avocados (and the oils made from them) are both rich sources of MUFAs. Nuts, canola oil, sunflower oil and safflower oil also provide dietary MUFA, and small amounts are found in lard. Monounsaturated fatty acids have been shown to decrease the risk of cardiovascular disease.

Polyunsaturated fatty acids (PUFAs) are found in oily fish, nuts, seeds and oils such as canola, sunflower, safflower, corn and soybean. Including PUFAs in your diet has been shown to decrease the risk of cardiovascular disease.

Of course, it's not quite as simple as this. Unsaturated fats also get divided into 'omega' families. The omega number indicates where on the chain of carbons the first double bond is found. So, omega-3 fatty acids have the first double bond on the third carbon atom from the end of the chain. Omega-6 fatty acids have the first double bond on the sixth carbon from the end, and so on. Humans can't make omega-3 or omega-6 fatty acids, so it's essential that we get them in our diet.

The dietary omegas that get most attention are omega-3 and omega-6, which are both PUFAs. It's recently been suggested that Western diets contain too much omega-6 and too little

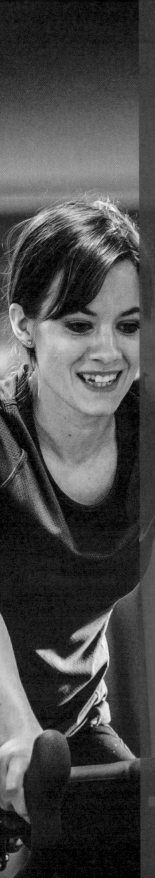

LOOK AFTER YOURSELF

Hannah, 38

I was pretty nervous about joining Nic's programme but I knew that I wanted to do something about my health. I was the heaviest I'd ever been and I found that I didn't have enough energy to juggle my family and work commitments.

I was quite relieved to find that his approach was a lot more balanced than I'd anticipated. I was already walking a few times a week, so I increased the frequency and duration of my walks – and it felt great, both mentally and physically. I added in a much more structured exercise programme that Nic designed, with some stretches and some bodyweight exercises.

I also used Nic's advice to help me change my diet – not drastically, but enough to make a difference. I focused on eating more lean protein, veges and fruit, and reducing carbs a bit.

I was surprised how just being aware of habits made it so much easier to change them – things like buying a chocolate bar at the check-out. I was also surprised at how much stress affected my eating. About a month or so into the programme I had a bit of a stressful time and I was intrigued to find myself craving chocolate for the first time since I'd started Nic's programme. But I was also happy to find that going for a walk cleared my head and left me feeling much better than if I'd given in to that craving.

The nice thing about this approach is that I don't feel guilty when special occasions come up and I eat 'celebration food'. I don't feel like I have to deny myself. I feel good, because most of the time I'm eating well.

Making some changes to my diet and exercise habits have had a big impact on my life. I've dropped a dress size and walked a half-marathon with ease. Most importantly, though, I've realised that I can justify taking the time to look after myself – it makes me a better mum and helps me cope with my job.

I'd definitely tell anyone thinking about using this approach to go for it! It will help you make realistic changes that you can sustain and that work for you and your life.

omega-3, and that this might contribute to chronic inflammation in the body. However, there doesn't yet appear to be any strong scientific evidence to support this, although research is continuing. It seems fair to say, though, that a diet containing a variety of fresh foods, including good sources of PUFAs, will be generally protective for health.

The importance of omega-3 fatty acids is not disputed. Diets high in oily fish are associated with much lower rates of cardiovascular disease. Since the initial finding was reported in the 1970s, researchers have looked at how effective omega-3 fatty acid supplements are for different groups of people; the results have mostly been positive. Omega-3 fatty acids are also thought to play a role in foetal brain development, and may alleviate some of the symptoms of people suffering from Alzheimer's disease.

The two omega-3 fatty acids that come from oily fish are eicosapentaenoic acid (EPA) and docosahexaenoic acid (DHA). Another omega-3, alpha-linolenic acid (ALA), comes from plants, particularly flax and chia seeds, walnuts, and canola and soybean oils. ALA is thought to be good for chronic inflammatory conditions such as rheumatoid arthritis, inflammatory bowel disease and metabolic syndrome.

There are two important omega fatty acids in the MUFA group – omega-9 and omega-7. The main omega-9 fatty acid in our food is oleic acid, which is found in olive oil and some animal fats. What's interesting is that in studies using oleic acid from animal fats, researchers don't see the same protection against heart disease that occurs when the omega-9 comes from olive oil. Your body can actually make its own omega-9 (provided that it gets the raw materials from your diet), so you don't need to consume it – but it's definitely not something to avoid, either!

Omega-7 fatty acids haven't been studied anywhere near as much as their -3, -6 and -9 cousins, but there's some evidence they may improve blood lipids and insulin resistance. Omega-7 fatty acids are found in macadamia nuts, meat and dairy foods.

BE CAREFUL WITH CANOLA

Canola oil is a popular choice for many people – it's affordable, it contains unsaturated fatty acids, and it's relatively flavourless, making it great for baking and cooking. However, a study in mice has shown it might not be totally healthy.

The researchers involved in this work had previously shown that including olive oil in the diet of laboratory mice had caused improvements in their memory and their brain structure. In particular, it had reduced levels of two substances that are increased in people suffering from Alzheimer's disease. The researchers were curious to see whether they could get the same effect from canola oil.

What they found was the opposite. After six months on a diet supplemented with canola oil, the mice had impaired memory function (this was measured using maze tests, as you can't ask a mouse if it can remember who the prime minister is). Not only that, but the brains of these mice were also changed, with fewer connections between neurons and more of the amyloid plaques that are associated with Alzheimer's. The mice were also heavier than their canola-free counterparts, even though both groups received the same balance of macronutrients in their diet.

Although this work was done with mice, not people, it still might be worth keeping your canola oil intake lower than your olive oil intake.

FATS IN THE FRIDGE (AND OTHER PLACES)

FAT SOURCE	FEATURES
Dairy (milk, butter, cheese)	These all contain saturated fat.
Olive oil	The top source of MUFAs, with 9.1 g in 1 tbsp of oil. Extra virgin also contains vitamins E and K and will have more antioxidants than more processed varieties.
Canola oil, sunflower oil, safflower oil	Good sources of MUFAs and PUFAs. 1 tbsp of canola oil contains 8 g of MUFA; 1 tbsp of sunflower oil contains 8.6 g of PUFA, while 1 tbsp of safflower oil contains 9 g of PUFA.
Oily fish (salmon, sardines, mackerel, herrings)	Oily fish are an excellent source of omega-3 fatty acids. 100 g of sardines supplies nearly 10 g of MUFA/PUFA. The same quantity of canned red salmon provides 5.2 g; smoked salmon provides 3.4 g and 100 g of tinned tuna in brine provides 1.8 g.
Red meat	Red meat contains both saturated and unsaturated fats, the latter mainly as MUFAs. A small grilled fillet steak contains 7.6 g of saturated fat, while a small grilled pork chop contains 3.8 g of saturated fat.
Chicken	Chicken is much lower in fat than other meats, and a greater proportion of the fat is MUFAs. A grilled chicken breast provides just under 5 g of fat, with half of that being MUFA.
Avocados (and avocado oil)	Avocado oil is great as it has a very high smoke point and so it doesn't break down and start burning as easily as other oils. It's almost all MUFA – 100 g of avocado oil contains around 76 g MUFA.
Nuts (and nut oils)	These mainly provide MUFAs, e.g. 100 g of almonds contains 55.6 g of fat, of which 68% is MUFA. Macadamias contain 74 g of fat, of which 79% is MUFA. 1 tbsp of peanut butter contains 6 g of fat, of which half is MUFA.
Seeds (and seed oils)	Seeds are excellent sources of unsaturated fats. A 100 g portion of pumpkin seeds contains around 44 g of fat, with 80% of that being MUFA/PUFA. Sunflower seeds are even higher in fat – a 100 g portion contains 47.4 g, with 90% of that being MUFA/PUFA.
Pastry, cakes, biscuits	These will be made with saturated fats, either butter or an oil that has been hydrogenated or partially hydrogenated to give it similar properties to butter.

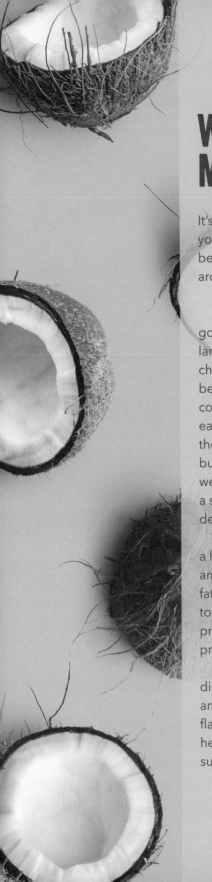

WILL COCONUT FAT MAKE ME THIN?

It's on Instagram, Pinterest and probably your Facebook feed, too. If all the hype is to be believed, coconut oil is the healthiest fat around and eating it will help you lose weight.

Unfortunately, the science doesn't stack up. Coconut oil is a highly saturated fat – it's got more saturated fat (92%!) than butter or lard. Most of this fat is present as medium-chain fatty acids, and this is where its health benefits are supposed to come from. A couple of studies have shown that people eating a concoction of pure MUFAs reduced their overall fat levels and appeared to burn fat more effectively. But these people weren't eating coconut oil – they were eating a supplement that had been specifically designed for the experiment.

Coconut oil has also been proposed as a heart-healthy fat because it contains high amounts of lauric acid – which is a saturated fatty acid that appears to alter the ratio of total cholesterol to HDL cholesterol. A greater proportion of HDL cholesterol is thought to protect against heart disease.

So, should you include coconut oil in your diet? It's certainly going to be safe in small amounts, especially if you're using it to add flavour to a dish and if you use it alongside healthy fats and oils, like olive, avocado and sunflower. But it's not going to make you thin!

#19 VITAMINS, MINERALS . . . AND PHYTONUTRIENTS

Carbohydrates, proteins and fats are all required in relatively large amounts for human health. Because they're needed in such large quantities, carbs, fat and protein are called **macronutrients** – 'macro' coming from the Greek word *makros*, meaning large.

In contrast, vitamins and minerals are required in tiny amounts, so are called **micronutrients** – 'micro' coming from the Greek word *mikros*, meaning small.

- # **Vitamins** are organic molecules, which means they contain carbon atoms. They are found in foods – either naturally in real foods or supplemented in some manufactured foods.
- # **Minerals** are inorganic – they don't contain carbon. Minerals are also found in food, and a few are added to manufactured products, sometimes to make up for naturally occurring deficiencies.

Then there are **phytonutrients**, which are organic substances found in plants. These help protect the plants from attacks by pests and diseases. Phytonutrients aren't essential for human health, but there's an increasing amount of evidence that they contribute to our wellbeing when consumed as part of a healthy diet.

VITAMINS

Vitamins are divided into two distinct groups – fat-soluble and water-soluble. The fat-soluble vitamins are A, D, E and K. These vitamins are absorbed into the body in the small intestine, and

INSIDE YOUR GUT

it's easier for your body to extract them from your food if there's also some fat present. A bit of butter on your carrots, for instance, improves the availability of vitamin A. Once in your body, these vitamins are stored in your fatty tissues. Because you can store these vitamins, it's not essential for you to get them in your food every day.

That's not the case for water-soluble vitamins, however. With these, anything you don't use leaves your body pretty quickly, which means that you need a regular supply for the best health. (The exception is vitamin B_{12}, which is stored in the liver.) The water-soluble vitamins include all members of the B group (B_1, B_2, B_3, B_5, B_6, B_7, B_9, B_{12}) and vitamin C.

Even though they are only needed in tiny amounts, vitamins are incredibly important to our health. They affect every part of our body, inside and out. Here's just a selection of the roles that they play:

   # Vitamin A – important for skin, bone and eye health. Also helps keep your mucous membranes healthy.

   # Vitamin B_1 (thiamine) – helps your body get energy from carbohydrates in your food and is also important for good nerve function.

   # Vitamin B_2 (riboflavin) – works with other B vitamins to maintain the production of red blood cells.

   # Vitamin B_3 (niacin) – required for skin and nerve health, red blood cell formation and the release of energy from carbohydrates in your food.

   # Vitamin B_5 (pantothenic acid) – needed for the breakdown of carbohydrate, fat and protein in your food, and plays a part in the production of a range of fats, hormones and neurotransmitters.

   # Vitamin B_6 – helps your body make and alter amino acids, which can then be used for cell growth or metabolism; also required for a healthy nervous system.

   # Vitamin B_7 (biotin) – works with other B vitamins to extract energy and nutrition from your food.

   # Vitamin B_9 (folic acid) – helps to maintain the DNA in your cells, and is also needed for the production of some neurotransmitters, such as serotonin.

Vitamin B_{12} – needed for the formation of the myelin sheath around nerves, and is also essential for cell division.
Vitamin C (ascorbic acid) – required for the formation of collagen; is the main protein in connective tissue.
Vitamin D – required for the formation of bones and teeth, and also helps maintain a healthy nerve and muscle system.
Vitamin E (tocopherol) – a powerful antioxidant that protects tissues against damage.
Vitamin K – helps regulate normal blood clotting functions.

These are by no means all the roles that vitamins play in your body, but it should be enough to show you just how essential it is to eat a diet that provides these micronutrients.

MINERALS

If you reduced a human body to its basics, you'd end up with a lot of carbon, hydrogen, oxygen and nitrogen, and a pile of assorted minerals. Those minerals include calcium, phosphorus, magnesium, potassium, sulphur, sodium and chloride, which together form the majority of our little pile. There are also small amounts of a wide range of other minerals – boron, cobalt, copper, fluoride, iodine, iron, manganese, selenium, zinc and more.

All of these minerals play a role in keeping your body healthy – either because they are part of the structure of your cells, or because they're involved in the various metabolic reactions that go on every minute of your life. Here are some of the many roles of some important vitamins:

Boron – required for building strong, healthy bones. It is most abundant in fruits, vegetables and nuts.
Cobalt – needed for the formation of vitamin B_{12}. It is most usefully found in animal-based foods, as there it's already in the form of vitamin B_{12}. Cobalt is also present in fruits and vegetables, but not in the form of B_{12}.

Copper – essential for the development and maintenance of the cardiovascular and nervous systems, and helps with iron absorption. Copper is present in many foods, although it is low in dairy products.
Fluoride – increases the strength of teeth and bones. It mainly comes from fluoridated water, and from plants grown in soil that contains fluoride.
Iodine – a component of thyroid hormones, which regulate metabolism and growth. It's mainly found in seafood and iodised salt.
Iron – mainly used as the central component of haemoglobin, the oxygen-carrying substance in our red blood cells. Dietary iron comes from meats, dried fruit, legumes, dark green leafy vegetables and prune juice.
Manganese – is involved in the formation of various tissues, including connective tissue, bone, proteins and blood clotting factors. It is provided by spinach, tea, whole grains, legumes, nuts and some fruits.
Selenium – an antioxidant, and also important as part of an enzyme that protects red blood cells against damage. It's found in grains that were grown in selenium-rich soil and also in meats.
Zinc – plays multiple roles in human health, including the detoxification of alcohol in the liver, wound healing and the functioning of insulin. Good sources include oysters, lean meat, poultry and fish. Wholegrain bread and cereals also provide some zinc.

As this selection of minerals shows, your body requires a range of nutrients in order to function well. The best way to achieve this is to eat a varied diet full of fresh food – or, at least, food that has not been deconstructed and then rebuilt into long-life items that fit neatly into a cardboard box!

PHYTONUTRIENTS

Phytonutrients are compounds that occur naturally in plants – in green, leafy vegetables, root vegetables and brightly coloured fruits, and in nuts, seeds and grains. Within the plant they help to prevent disease, reduce the likelihood of attack by pests, and protect against sun damage. There are literally thousands of phytonutrients – more than 25,000 different compounds have been identified so far. It's quite possible that some of these have absolutely no impact on human health, but others definitely do have strong, beneficial effects. Here are some of the most commonly discussed phytonutrients:

Beta-carotene – found in yellow and orange fruits and vegetables, most notably carrots, this helps maintain healthy eyes. When you eat beta-carotene, it is converted into vitamin A in your small intestine.

Lycopene – found in red fruits, most famously in tomatoes. Lycopene has powerful antioxidant effects and appears to help protect against the development of some cancers.

Lutein and zeaxanthin – these dominate in yellow vegetables such as sweetcorn, and dark green leafy vegetables such as spinach, silverbeet and kale. Both appear to offer protection against eye disorders associated with ageing, such as cataracts and macular degeneration.

Ellagic acid – found in strawberries, raspberries and pomegranates, it may help your liver neutralise cancer-promoting compounds.

Glucosinolates – that bitter flavour you can taste in broccoli, Brussels sprouts and cabbage is down to the glucosinolates they contain. It's good, though, as these compounds appear to check the development of cancer cells.

Phytoestrogens – these compounds act a bit like oestrogen. Key sources are soy products (which supply isoflavones) and flax and sesame seeds (which supply lignans). There's some evidence that women who include

some soy in their diet have a lower risk of endometrial cancer and bone loss.

\# Resveratrol – this shot to fame when it was proposed as the reason why the French had lower rates of heart disease despite consuming a lot of animal fat. Resveratrol, which is found in the skins of red grapes (and therefore in red wine), was thought to be the protective agent involved, and studies do show that it appears to reduce the risk of coronary heart disease.

\# Catechins – these compounds are found in green tea and may help to reduce the risk of cancer cells developing.

\# Quercetin – found in several fruit and vegetables, including apples and onions, quercetin may help reduce the risk of asthma and heart disease.

\# Curcumin – another phytonutrient much discussed these days, it's found in high amounts in turmeric. However, it's been difficult to conclusively show what effects this has in the body, because of the way it behaves in experiments.

Of course, we humans tend to think that if a small amount of something is good, then a big amount of it must be so much better. This is what supports the supplements industry! If you eat a healthy diet, then you won't need supplements. Save your money for buying seasonal fresh vegetables and fruit – you'll get phytonutrients in their natural, unprocessed state, and you'll get a wide range of them rather than a single isolated compound.

DID YOU KNOW?

You can actually change the colour of your skin if you eat too much beta-carotene. It's temporary, though – the yellow-orange colour fades when you reduce your beta-carotene intake to more normal levels.

#20 THINKIN' 'BOUT DRINKIN'

You'll no doubt have heard that you need to drink eight glasses of water a day to stay hydrated. You might also have heard that there's absolutely no scientific evidence to back up this claim. In fact, one study has shown that men typically require 3.7 litres of fluid a day and women need 2.7 litres.

There's no doubt that you need to take in fluid each day to stay well hydrated, but how much you need depends on several factors – including the environment and your activity levels. If you go out for a 100 km bike ride on a stinking hot day, you'd better be upping your fluid intake!

On a regular day, some of your fluid intake will come from the food you eat, and the rest from drinking liquids. Some fruits and vegetables are almost straight water, held together with a bit of fibre, along with some fructose and a few minerals, vitamins and phytonutrients. Watermelon is a great example of this, which is why a slice is so refreshing on a hot day. Lettuce is a good example of a high-water vegetable.

Being well hydrated has a number of health advantages:
For a start, you feel better!
You'll probably also look better, because your skin will be plump and soft rather than dry and rough.
Your joints will thank you. Joints contain synovial fluid, which cushions them and helps them move freely. When you're well hydrated, you'll have enough fluid to ensure that your synovial fluid levels are optimal – plus, this will help your body remove waste products from your joint spaces.
You'll be able to maintain your body temperature more easily. This is particularly important in hot weather, when you need to be able to sweat in order to cool down – if

you're dehydrated, your body will reduce sweating to conserve fluid.

\# Liquid waste removal is more effective. When you're properly hydrated, your blood volume is higher, and this means that your blood will move more easily through your veins, arteries and capillaries. In turn, this means that it reaches your kidneys more easily so that they can extract the waste products (as well as receiving the nutrients they need to function).

\# Solid waste removal is more effective. A well-hydrated body is much less likely to suffer from constipation than one that's short on water. Undigested food and fibre in your lower colon is bulked up by water – and the bulkier it is, the easier it moves!

HELP WITH HYDRATION

The first sign that you're dehydrated is normally thirst. If you're thirsty, you need to take on some water. The problem is that a lot of us aren't that good at recognising thirst – we often think we're hungry when in fact our bodies are crying out for liquid.

A second reliable sign of dehydration is dark-coloured urine. If you're well hydrated, your urine will be a pale yellow colour (unless you've been eating beetroot, in which case it could have a pinkish tinge, or you've taken a multi-vitamin containing riboflavin – vitamin B_2 – which will turn your urine bright yellow).

Although short-term dehydration won't kill you, prevention is still better than cure. Drinking regularly during the day will help keep you hydrated – unless you interpret 'drinking' as meaning alcoholic drinks! Alcohol will dehydrate you (see page 163).

WHAT TO DRINK – AND WHAT NOT TO

\# The best fluid you can drink is water. Tap water is free, and in most countries it's safe to drink. Bottled water is OK, too, if you prefer (although the packaging isn't that great for the environment).

- # Tea is good, as long as you don't add sugar. Regular, green, flavoured, herbal, fruit – there are lots of options so you can mix it up a bit.

- # Coffee is a diuretic – it makes you want to urinate – but it doesn't cause you to lose more fluid than you've drunk. Some is OK, but it's best not to overdo it.

- # Sugar-free fizzy drinks (soda water and diet drinks) are OK, but some of them might not be that good for your teeth. This particularly applies to drinks that are cola-based or fruit-based, since these tend to be more acidic – they can weaken your tooth enamel if you drink them regularly. Some people prefer not to consume artificial sweeteners, and it's generally going to be better for you to wean yourself off sweet flavours, whether artificial or natural.

- # Fruit juice and sugary fizzy drinks are a definite no-no. Both contain high levels of sugars (fructose, glucose, sucrose) that you don't need in your diet on a regular basis. It doesn't matter whether the sugar comes from cane sugar, coconut sugar, high-fructose corn syrup or any other type of sweetener – it's still going to end up as glucose in your bloodstream.

A glass of water first thing in the morning is a great way to start the day. If you want to add a splash of lemon juice or apple cider vinegar (see page 167), that's up to you – but don't do it because you think it's going to offer you any magical health benefits. And maybe have a chat with your dentist first, as acidic drinks can erode your tooth enamel.

During the day, keep topped up with water. Green tea, herbal teas, black tea and black coffee in moderation are OK, too. Sports drinks are not a good choice for most people – you have to be doing an awful lot of manual labour or hard-core exercise to need the electrolytes – and sugar! – in these drinks.

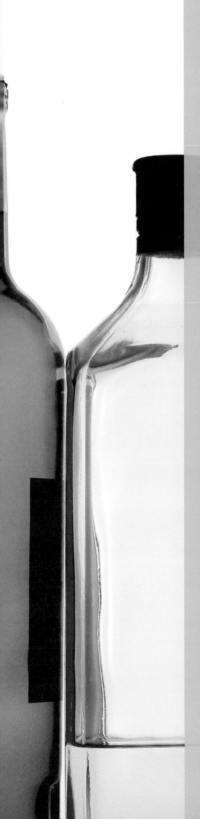

DRYING OUT WITH ALCOHOL

If you drink alcohol, then you'll end up losing more fluid than you take in. How does this happen? It's because of the effect of alcohol on a substance called vasopressin, which is produced by the pituitary gland in your brain.

If you're dehydrated, your pituitary gland pumps out more vasopressin, which reduces the amount of urine you produce. You'll hold on to more of the water in your body so that you don't become even more dehydrated.

Alcohol completely upends this process. It makes your pituitary gland reduce vasopressin production, so now you'll start to produce greater amounts of urine. You'll end up pumping out much more liquid than you've drunk.

A standard alcoholic drink contains 10 g of alcohol. This amount will cause your body to produce an extra 120 ml of urine, over and above the amount you'd normally make. Even if you drink extra water alongside your alcohol of choice, you'll probably still end up more dehydrated than when you started out!

#21 SO, WHAT SHOULD I EAT?

THE BIG 10

THIS IS ALL IT TAKES:

- # Eat fresh, natural foods.
- # Eat a rainbow every day.
- # Reduce the amount of white foods you eat.
- # Be aware of portion sizes.
- # Stay well hydrated.
- # Keep fruit intake moderate.
- # Reduce your alcohol intake.
- # Be prepared.
- # Be organised.
- # Be consistent.

A few generations ago, people knew what food was, and in most cases, it consisted of plants, meat, eggs and dairy. Meals were made at home, as were baked goods like scones, biscuits and puddings. Today, all of those foods are still there – but they've been joined by an ever-increasing number of commercially manufactured items. As a result, for many of us food consists of things that come in cardboard boxes, whether off the shelf or out of the chiller.

Not only that, but we eat out a lot more these days. Whether it's Sunday brunch at a café, mid-week coffee and cake with friends, a work-day lunch from a sandwich bar, Friday-night fish and chips or an any-time meal at the food court at the local mall, opportunities for eating out are everywhere!

This rapid change in our eating environment has left many of us out of touch with traditional foods. Half the time we wouldn't have a clue what's gone into our meals, let alone what sort of

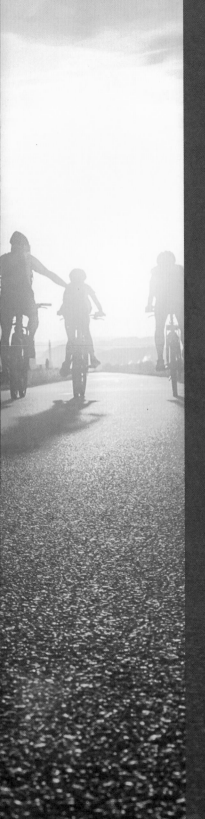

FIT:5

Real food for the real you

Eating doesn't have to be complicated. Follow these five tips, and you'll be getting all the macronutrients, micronutrients and fibre that you need to stay healthy.

1. Base your meals around lean protein - red meat, chicken, fish, eggs, beans, nuts, soy products; whatever you prefer.
2. Add loads of vegetables - you can use fresh, frozen, or even canned, provided that they don't have added sugar.
3. Choose colourful vegetables over white ones, and eat more above-ground than root vegetables.
4. Limit your fruit consumption to two pieces a day, max - and eat it fresh and whole, not as juice.
5. Drink water. Tea, coffee and green tea are good, too, as long as you don't add sugar. Avoid all sweetened drinks.

nutritional value they offer. We're wandering blind and bloated through a land filled with salt, sugar and fat.

Fortunately, it doesn't have to be this way. You can reclaim control of your diet and get your health back by following a few simple guidelines. Yes, it will take more effort to start with – but as you progress, you'll become more skilled at building healthy meals, and you'll have more energy for this, as well as all of the other activities you enjoy. OK, so it might look a lot – but in reality, it's not. Most of these steps are relatively easy to achieve, and the following sections will show you how.

APPLE CIDER VINEGAR

There are plenty of diet gurus around who would just about stake their lives on the all-encompassing benefits of apple cider vinegar. It's said to do all sorts of things, from helping you lose weight to curing a sore throat or even varicose veins! Sadly, there isn't much scientific evidence for most of these claims.

A few small studies have looked at the effect of apple cider vinegar on blood sugar control. In one study, 10 men with type 1 diabetes drank either 30 ml apple cider vinegar (mixed with 20 ml water) or 50 ml water. Five minutes later, they all ate an identical, high-carbohydrate meal. The men's blood glucose levels were measured over the following 4 hours. For the first 30 minutes, the rise in blood glucose was the same in both groups, but after that it rose much more slowly in the men who'd received the vinegar; and it didn't get to the same peak level as it did in the men who had drunk just water.

A similar study looked at the effect of apple cider vinegar on normal (insulin-sensitive), pre-diabetic (insulin-resistant) and type 2 diabetic people. Again, the study was small, only involving 29 people altogether. Each person consumed 20 g of apple cider vinegar and then ate a high-carbohydrate meal within the next 2 minutes. The vinegar produced lower blood glucose and blood insulin levels in all of the test groups, with the strongest effect being seen in those people who were insulin-resistant.

What might be happening? Well, vinegar is known to slow the rate at which the stomach empties, and it also suppresses the activity of a couple of enzymes that help break down carbohydrate. These might be part of the reason for its effects.

Does apple cider vinegar have a role in a healthy lifestyle? Well, it probably won't do you any harm (provided that you don't let it slosh all over your teeth) – but it's not going to magically reverse the effects of an unhealthy diet. If you do want to try it, remember that you need to eat a high-carbohydrate meal straight afterwards to get any benefit.

#22 EAT FRESH, EAT NATURAL

Where do you shop for your food? If you're like most people, you do the majority of your food shopping at a supermarket. And once you're in that shop, you quite unwittingly give up a bit of your free choice.

Supermarkets are designed to make you part with your money. From the moment you walk in the door to the time you pay at the checkout, everything is engineered to get you to buy. Before you even get inside the doors, there are the shopping trolleys – see how huge they are? That's to encourage you to put more inside them. Now the fruit and veg section – an expanse of colour, the minute you get inside. You'll no doubt pick up some produce here and feel like you're off on the right foot. And that's exactly what the supermarket gurus want you to think.

So then you round the corner and see the wine, and you think how nice a bottle would be with that lovely fresh food you've picked up. Go on, get one – oh, look, this one's on special. Might as well get a couple, then.

Now you're on a roll, moving up and down the aisles – but slowly, because the tempo of the background music is making sure that you cruise through, not dash through. And the eye-catching displays make you stop frequently – either because you can't find what you're looking for, or because you spot something new on the shelves. The ends of the aisles aren't hazard-free zones, either. Quite the opposite – they're packed full of promotions, because even if you're not going to go down a particular aisle you'll still walk past the end of it. Specials, super-specials, buy one, get one free deals – they're all designed to get you to buy more.

By the time you reach the chilled and frozen section, you're tired and worn out, and the smell of freshly baked bread has made you hungry. Making dinner suddenly seems like far too much work, so you pick up a couple of frozen pizzas instead. Hey, the Italians have wine and pizza all the time, don't they? Must be part of that healthy Mediterranean diet . . .

It doesn't stop at the checkout, either. Even 'candy-free' checkouts are still stashed with snacks for those last-minute spontaneous purchases.

And notice how there are no clocks on display, so you're not really aware of how long you've been in the shop?

By the time you come out, you've usually bought a lot more than you bargained for – and a lot of that will be processed and in boxes and not designed to give you optimal health.

TAKE CONTROL OF YOUR SHOPPING

So, can you eat fresh and natural and still shop at a supermarket? Yes, absolutely. The trick is to shop the perimeter, and avoid going into the aisles unless they have a specific ingredient that you absolutely must buy – olive oil or tinned fish, for instance.

If you stay outside the aisles, you'll be able to buy fresh fruit and veges, fish, meat, dairy, eggs and most likely nuts and seeds, too. The bakery is also on that path, but unless you've got a will of steel you're best to just look away.

Take a shopping list with you, and don't go to the supermarket when you're hungry. This isn't groundbreaking advice, but so few of us do it! You can write a list on a piece of paper, or you can go the tech route and get an app for your phone – OurGroceries is a good one, and it lets you set up lists for different stores.

Another option is not to go to the supermarket at all. Do your shopping online and have it delivered to you. That way, you avoid the temptation of marked-down bakery products and two-for-one deals on potato chips. Yes, there's usually a delivery fee – but think about how much you could save this way: the cost of the petrol (assuming that you're making a special trip and not just calling in on the way home), the cost of your time (and that's worth plenty!) and the cost of all of those spontaneous purchases that you really didn't need.

You could also decide to bypass supermarkets altogether. If you're lucky enough to have a good fruit and vege shop, a

HOW DENSE IS THAT?

As a rule, fresh, natural foods are nutrient-dense. This means that each portion of the food delivers a lot of health value because relative to the number of calories it has, it contains a high proportion of vitamins, minerals, fibre, protein or good fats. The opposite of this is calorie-dense food. Foods in this category contain a lot of calories but little in the way of nutrients that your body can use for anything other than energy.

To see the difference, take a look at the table opposite, which compares silverbeet with white bread. First, we've compared the nutrient value of 100 g of each of these. Then, since white bread has 10 times the calories of silverbeet, we've also shown the nutrient value delivered by 10 g of white bread, which has the same number of calories as 100 g of silverbeet. Just for interest, a slice of white bread usually weighs around 30 g.

Even without accounting for the calorie difference between the two foods, silverbeet wins out nutritionally on seven of the nutrient measurements. When we take the calories into account, silverbeet is not only higher in fibre but it's also nutritionally better on an additional five measurements and equivalent on one more (thiamine). The only nutrient that is more abundant in bread is selenium, and that is most likely because wheat crops are grown in soil that has selenium added to it in order to boost the selenium content of the grain used for milling.

By choosing nutrient-dense foods, you'll be super-charging your diet and making sure that your body gets all the nutrition it needs to be healthy, without being weighed down by too many unnecessary calories.

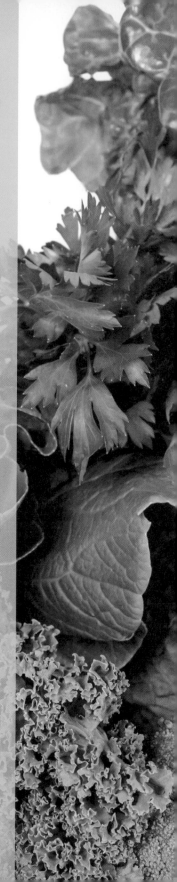

bakery, a butchery, a fishmonger and a delicatessen within a reasonable distance of your home or work, then you could decide to support those stores and just visit the supermarket occasionally.

There is no single solution that's going to work for everyone – and probably no single solution that will work for you all the time. Experiment. Try a different approach each week. See what you like and what you don't like. And then build your own portfolio of shopping tactics that will help you choose fresh, natural food that supports your health and fitness.

NUTRIENT	100 G SILVERBEET	100 G WHITE BREAD	10 G WHITE BREAD
Calories	25 calories	251 calories	25 calories
Fibre	3.3 g	5.6 g	0.56 g
Potassium	421 mg	101 mg	10.1 mg
Phosphorus	39 mg	78 mg	7.8 mg
Calcium	68 mg	19 mg	1.9 mg
Iron	1.2 mg	6 mg	0.6 mg
Zinc	0.7 mg	0.8 mg	0.08 mg
Selenium	0.3 µg	3.6 µg	0.36 µg
Vitamin A equivalent	553 µg	0	0
Beta-carotene equivalent	3310 µg	0	0
Thiamine	0.02 mg	0.22 mg	0.02 mg
Riboflavin	0.04 mg	0.05 mg	0.005 mg
Niacin equivalent	0.9 mg	2.3 mg	0.23 mg
Vitamin B_6	0.25 mg	0.05 mg	0.005 mg
Vitamin B_{12}	0	0	0
Folate B_9	49 µg	22 µg	2.2 µg
Vitamin C	16 mg	0	0
Vitamin D	0	0	0

* Data from The Concise New Zealand Food Composition Tables, 2009

#23 EAT A RAINBOW

Colour is the key to good health. And that colour's not white - or brown. No, a healthy diet is full of green and orange and red and purple. It's not quite a rainbow, but it's not a sand dune either! Many of us eat a pretty restricted diet, and we could get a lot of health benefits from expanding that.

If the only veg you normally eat are frozen peas and frozen sweetcorn, where do you start? Let's take a look at your options:

Green - asparagus, avocado, bok choy, broad beans, broccoli, Brussels sprouts, cabbage, celery, cucumber, edamame beans, fennel, green beans, green capsicum, kale, leeks, lettuce, microgreens, okra, peas, rocket, sugar snap peas, spinach, silverbeet, spring onion, watercress, zucchini.

Orange - orange capsicum, carrots, pumpkin, butternut, yams.

Red - tomatoes, red capsicum, kumara, red onions, radishes, yams, radicchio.

Purple - purple carrots, eggplant, beetroot, kumara, purple potatoes, purple asparagus, red cabbage, purple capsicum.

Yellow - yellow capsicum, yellow beetroot, yellow carrots, yams, sweetcorn, yellow tomatoes, yellow sweet potato.

OK - that should give you something to start with!

Now, of course you don't have to eat a rainbow at every meal. Unless you have a personal chef, you'd spend far too long in the kitchen. But you should aim to eat a rainbow through the day and through the week. (Although if you *could* shoot for the stars and have loads of colour at every meal, that would be outstanding!)

This doesn't have to be an expensive exercise, either. If you use frozen vegetables and add in some fresh veg that's in

GREEN GOODNESS

Want to preserve your brain function so that you can still think straight when you're older? Eating greens might just be what you need. A study in the United States found that people who ate one serving of leafy greens every day retained their thinking and memory skills better than people who hardly ever ate greens. The study involved elderly volunteers with an average age of 81, and ran for 10 years. Those who ate hardly any green veg had a much greater decline in mental function – so much so that by the end of the experiment they were an average 11 years older, cognitively, than the green vege eaters! It just goes to show that you're never too young to benefit from some healthy eating.

season, then you've got an affordable rainbow. Do a little check when you're in the supermarket – has your trolley got a rainbow of colour from the fruit and veg section?

When you're thinking about what veges to eat, try to focus more on those that grow above the ground than on root vegetables.

Root veges are storage vessels for plants, which means that they're generally higher in calories and starch or sugars than veges that grow above the ground.
Vegetables that grow above the ground tend to contain more phytonutrients, because they need them to reduce the chance of attack from insects and pests.

There's no need to eliminate root veg from your diet – especially the more colourful ones like carrots and beetroot and sweet potato. It's just a matter of keeping them in balance with the rest of the food on your plate.

#24 WHERE THE WHITE STUFF HIDES

How many servings of white food do you eat in a day? One? Five? Ten? If no one's ever asked before, then you're probably fairly oblivious to how much white food you eat. And this matters – because, for the most part, white food is not healthy food. Often, it's just bulk. It's calories without much in the way of nutritional value.

Unfortunately, white food is also easy and convenient. Here's a selection of common foods that shows just how pervasive it is in a modern diet.

Bread: white, brown, wholemeal, sliced, sourdough, wraps, rolls – it really doesn't matter. These are all essentially white – they're made with grains that have been finely ground, which means that they are incredibly easy for your body to digest. Yes, a sourdough wholegrain loaf with added seeds will be better for you than a slice of mass-market white, but the gains are relatively small.

Crackers: wheat-based, rice-based, flavoured or plain – they are all essentially the same. Like bread, they are made from grains that have been finely ground, and for the most part they offer little nutritional value.

Cakes and biscuits: a double-whammy of white – these contain both white flour and sugar! Fine as a treat; no good at all as a fundamental building block of your daily diet.

Pasta: white, wholemeal, gluten-free – and it doesn't matter what shape it is! Pasta is a great carrier for meat-

or vegetable-based sauces, but meals often have huge quantities of it, which just piles on the calories.

\# Rice: on the side, in sushi, in a risotto, under a curry – like pasta, rice often plays a far too dominant role in many meals.

\# Potatoes: baked, mashed, roasted, boiled – yes, potatoes do offer some nutrients, especially if the skin is eaten. However, all too often they are just bulk filling up the plate – and there are better ways to do this.

\# Pies, pastries and pizzas – all common quick-fix foods, all full of white flour and usually containing a load of saturated fat to further damage your health.

\# Sausages, sausage rolls and similar goods – if it's got pastry, it's got flour. If it's a cheap sausage, it will undoubtedly have bread in it as a filler; the more expensive sausages are more likely to be mainly meat.

\# Commercial breakfast cereals – the boxes may be loaded with colour, but the contents generally aren't (at least, not in a nutritionally good way). Most (but not all) commercial breakfast cereals mainly contain grains that have been milled and reshaped to appeal to our eyes and they contain lots of sugar.

If you want to improve your health, then minimising the amount of white food in your diet is a great step. The reason? It creates a big space where you can put foods that have much more nutritional value – high-quality proteins that your body can use to restore and build your tissues, healthy fats to keep your cells supple, colourful vegetables and fruits that are full of vitamins, minerals and phytonutrients to help keep you young (or at least to stop you ageing so fast!).

WHAT, SO NO BREAD EVER AGAIN?

Watching out for the white stuff doesn't mean giving it up forever – that would be a sure-fire road to failure. The trick is to reduce the amount that you routinely eat, and to mix up your diet so that you're getting more variety.

Let's say dinner was going to be a nice piece of baked fish, a jacket potato, some broccoli, some green beans and some sweetcorn, and you were going to round that off with some garlic bread. That meal's got two types of white food – the potato and the garlic bread. If you've had a really active day, then you might be able to get away with eating both. If you've had a moderately active day, then instead of having both, just have one – you get to choose which one. And if you've had a really sedentary day, you'd be better off leaving both off your plate and adding some more vegetables to fill the gap.

This is the 'earn it or burn it' approach. If you think of your body as a car, then carbs are the petrol. (Proteins, fats, vitamins, minerals and phytonutrients are the oil, transmission fluid, brake fluid, etc.) If your car's doing lots of travel, you need lots of petrol. It's the same with your body: if you've done lots of physical activity in the day, then you'll have earned your calories. Ideally, most of these calories will come from good-quality, nutritious foods – but some of them can certainly come from foods that mainly supply energy. What foods those are depend on your tastes. For some people it's going to be bread, for others it could be ice cream, for others it could be a glass of red wine.

The flip side of this is the 'burn it' part – this means that you need to commit to using the calories you've already consumed. Did you go out to a café for brunch and have The Big Breakfast, with toast and hash browns alongside eggs, sausages, tomatoes and mushrooms? Then you'll probably need to get physical in the afternoon.

If you don't normally exercise in the second half of the day, this is a really difficult approach – you're using a stick, not a carrot. There's a strong chance that exercising in the afternoon is going to feel more like punishment for what you've done, whereas the 'earn it' approach frames your meal as a reward for your exercise effort. Be careful, too, that you don't start thinking 'Oh, I've been for a 20-minute run, so I'm fine to eat a large pizza, garlic bread and an ice cream.' You'll end up taking in way more energy than you used on the run. Use an app like MyFitnessPal to get an idea of how much energy you're expending and how much you're eating, and then use this information to guide your own food and exercise choices.

#25 HOW MUCH SHOULD I EAT?

Portion sizes have increased so dramatically over the past few decades that most of us haven't got a clue about how much we should eat for breakfast, lunch or dinner. This 'portion distortion' appears to have started with the fast-food industry – these businesses realised that they could increase the size of a meal at very little cost, charge more for it and still appear to be offering a bargain. It reached its climax with the 'super-size me' phenomenon, which was eventually halted in 2004 after negative public reaction to the documentary film *Super Size Me*.

However, you still have the option to buy large portions, and they still appear to be much better value than the smaller portions. A small fries from McDonald's is 231 calories, and a large fries is 405 – but the price difference doesn't reflect this so it could almost be regarded as sensible to choose the larger option. A small cola drink is 230 ml, the large is 500 – more than double the calories unless it's a sugar-free option. There's nothing special about McDonald's, either – these sorts of practices occur everywhere, and not just in the big-brand fast-food chains. Here are some other examples of oversized foods:

Muffins – at one time, these were cupcakes or fairy cakes. They were pretty small, and maybe took four or five delicate bites to eat. Now, they are massive. A double chocolate muffin from Muffin Break comes in at 166 g and delivers 633 calories (plus 5.1 g of fibre – so there's *some* good news).

Scones – in the past, scones were something your mother or grandmother whipped up when visitors turned up, and they typically measured 5–6 cm in diameter. Now, go into a café and it's not uncommon to see scones that are 15 cm in diameter.

Toasted sandwiches – these used to consist of two slices of bread with a bit of cheese and something else (tomato/pineapple/onion – pick your pleasure). Now, lots of places serve a toasted sandwich that consists of three slices of bread, each glued to the other with filling.

Chocolate bars – not content with offering us portable, affordable treats, chocolate companies have provided us with several ways to eat more of these goodies. First we had the 'king-sized' bar, then we had the 'twin-pack' – the idea being that we'd share this (yeah, right). We can also buy a share-pack of mini-sized treats. Although this might not be seen as oversizing, it encourages over-consumption because each little treat is so more-ish that once you start, it's hard to stop. And there's a whole bag of them.

Potato chips – while you can still buy small individual packs, larger sizes dominate the supermarket shelves. Those large packs are meant to be shared – but it's pretty easy for one person to eat most of a pack. Sizes have increased, too: a single pack of this type of snack food used to be 30 g; now it's often 40 g. Years ago, a party-size offering was three 100 g packs in a cardboard box – now we're regularly given the chance to buy three 150 g packs for $4, which makes a single 40 g pack look like a waste of money.

Fizzy drinks – the size increase here is similar to that for potato chips: small sizes are still available, but large sizes dominate the market. As a result, we're conditioned to buying much larger quantities. Sadly, it's all too common to see children and younger adults walking around with 1.25-litre bottles of fizzy drink.

And it's not just fast foods that have grown in size. In the 1980s, a typical dinner plate in the US was 25 cm in diameter; by the 2000s it was 30 cm, providing an extra 44% of plate that could be filled with food. This has also happened in Australia, New Zealand, the UK and probably many other countries, too. What used to be regarded as a dinner plate is now called a side plate.

There is some evidence that larger plate sizes encourage larger portion sizes. This would be fine if the extra space on the plate was taken up with low-calorie, nutrient-dense vegetables – but too often it's filled up with rice, potatoes or pasta.

MAKE-UP OF A MEAL

What does a good meal look like? Ideally, it will contain a mix of lean protein, colourful vegetables, something that delivers healthy fats, and some carbohydrate if needed. Now the question is how much of each of these types of food you should eat.

Traditional approaches to portion control tend to focus on calorie counting. 'You need X calories of protein, Y calories of fat, Z calories of carbohydrate.' It's good to have a general idea of the energy density of your food, but counting calories is a bit soul-destroying and for most people it takes away from the pleasure of eating.

An alternative approach is to use volume. You *could* measure out a cup of this and a half-cup of that – but there's an easier way, and that's to use the size of your hands as a guide. The advantage here is that the size of your hands is in proportion to the size of your body – this means that if you're 2 metres tall, you'll have a bit more food on your plate than if you're only 1.6 metres, which makes up for the extra energy you need to run a bigger body.

The other advantage of using your hands as a guide is that they are always with you. Eating out? Use your hands as a guide to how much you should be eating – regardless of the size of meal served up.

HANDS GUIDELINE

For each meal:
  # Lean protein – one palm-sized portion for red meat or chicken; one flat hand for white fish.
  # Non-starchy vegetables – two cupped handfuls, or more if you like.
  # Carb-dense foods – one cupped handful.
  # Fat-dense foods – one thumb-sized portion.

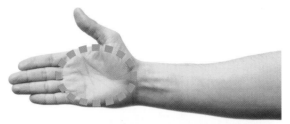

1 PALM OF RED MEAT OR CHICKEN

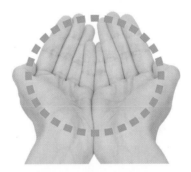

2 CUPPED HANDFULS OF NON-STARCHY VEGE

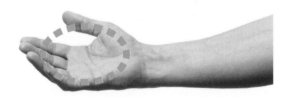

1 CUPPED HANDFUL OF CARBS

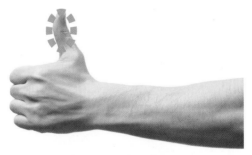

1 THUMB OF FAT

DESIGN YOUR PLATE

The other way is to design your plate so that about half of it contains non-starchy vegetables, about a fifth of it is whole grains, starchy vegetables or beans, a fifth is protein and just a tenth of the plate contains some healthy fats, like avocado or oily fish. This is a very easy, practical way to look at a meal, and can be applied to virtually any situation.

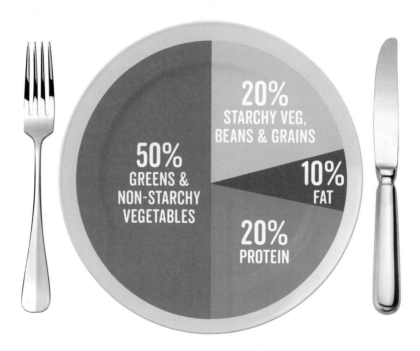

ADAPT AS NEEDED

Now, these examples are general guidelines only. Adapt them to your particular situation. Here are some examples:

- # **You're feeling really hungry:** First, add extra non-starchy vegetables – you can easily double the amount on your plate. If you still need more, opt for extra protein before adding extra carbs.
- # **You're trying to lose weight:** Leave the carbs off the plate, and add extra vegetables. If you really want to have some carbs, trying halving the amount on your plate.
- # **You're trying to gain weight:** Increase the amount of everything on your plate.
- # **You're trying to gain muscle:** Increase the amount of protein and non-starchy vegetables on your plate.
- # **You've had a carb-heavy breakfast:** Leave carbs out of your lunch and dinner, or at least reduce the quantity. Add extra vegetables to make up the volume.
- # **You've had a very physically active day:** Increase the amount of everything on your plate.
- # **You're going out for dinner tonight:** Don't eat any carbs at breakfast or lunch. Stick to the nutrient-dense protein and veges, with a bit of good fat.

IT COSTS HOW MUCH?!

Often, we don't realise exactly how much energy is stored in foods that we eat every day. Some foods have a 'health halo' – we think they are good for us, but in fact they may be hurting our efforts to stay lean. The examples on the following page turn 'healthy' foods into their 'unhealthy' equivalents, and also show just how much exercise is needed to burn off that energy.

'HEALTHY' FOOD	CALORIES*	EQUIVALENT CALORIES SHOWN AS		AMOUNT OF RUNNING/ (WALKING) TO BURN THIS ENERGY**	
		CHOCOLATE	BEER	65 KG WOMAN	95 KG MAN
Smoothie, 500 ml, made with milk, fruit juice, fruit, yoghurt	180	34 g	480 ml	14 min (33 min)	10 min (23 min)
Fruit juice, 500 ml	220	42 g	593 ml	18 min (41 min)	12 min (28 min)
Muesli, sweetened, toasted, 1 cup	443	84 g	1194 ml	35 min (82 min)	24 min (56 min)
Bread, white or brown, 2 slices	166	32 g	450 ml	13 min (31 min)	9 min (21 min)
Rice, cooked, 1 cup	170	32 g	458 ml	14 min (31 min)	9 min (22 min)
Pasta, cooked, 250 g	325	62 g	876 ml	26 min (60 min)	18 min (41 min)
Banana, large	133	25 g	358 ml	11 min (25 min)	7 min (17 min)
Kiwifruit, green, 3	165	31 g	444 ml	13 min (31 min)	9 min (21 min)

* Will vary depending on ingredients. Equivalents are based on 100 g chocolate being 530 calories and 1 litre of beer being 371 calories.

** Assumes a running pace of 12 km per hour, or a very brisk walking pace of 6.5 km per hour; times in minutes (min) are rounded to the nearest minute.

THE FRUIT FACTOR

Fruit is generally regarded as being good for us - and it's certainly a lot better than processed foods like bars and biscuits. But just because something is good for you doesn't mean that you should eat vast, unlimited amounts of it. Whichever way you look at it, that's not part of a healthy, balanced diet.

Fruit does contain fibre and phytonutrients, but it also contains sugar. True, that sugar isn't absorbed into your body as quickly as the sugar you put in your tea, but it still delivers calories. So, if you're looking to manage your weight, then it's worth being aware that eating too much fruit could hurt your chances of success.

One or two pieces of fruit a day are fine - but if you find yourself snacking on 10 kiwifruit each day, then you'll be eating a massive 550 calories, which is a big chunk of your daily needs. Bananas - our favourite fruit - are around 150 calories each, which is about the same as two chocolate digestives or Afghan biscuits. If you're aware that this is part of your energy intake and you adjust the rest of your diet to compensate, then maybe it will be OK. But most of us view fruit as 'free food', to be consumed without any consequences.

Try to keep fruit intake to two portions a day, and choose fruits that are highly coloured (blueberries, raspberries, oranges, plums, peaches) so that you get a good dose of phytonutrients at the same time.

A TALE OF TWO DIETS

Sometimes it's really obvious when a diet is unhealthy. If someone's eating burgers for breakfast, fried chicken for lunch, and pizza and beer for dinner every day, then they're probably not going to be the healthiest person on the planet.

But sometimes a diet *looks* healthy but isn't delivering the sort of nutritional punch you want. One reason for this is that we've been conditioned to eat a pretty narrow range of foods, and to eat certain types of foods at specific times. Hardly anyone thinks it's normal to eat vegetables at breakfast, for instance - but that's crazy: why shouldn't we eat veges at breakfast?

So, let's take a look at a 'healthy but conventional' day of eating, and compare it with a 'healthy but unconventional' day - and see how the nutrition stacks up for each of them.

CONVENTIONAL HEALTHY

Breakfast:
Muesli (1 cup), yoghurt (175 g), milk (½ cup), blueberries (¼ cup), glass of orange juice (250 ml)

Morning tea:
1 banana

Lunch:
Two sandwiches with egg and lettuce, 2 kiwifruit

Afternoon tea:
Small bag of nuts (50 g)

Dinner:
Steak (186 g), boiled potatoes (175 g), peas (40 g), broccoli (60 g)

Dessert:
Fruit salad (1 cup)

Looks pretty healthy, right? But dig deeper, and see all the white food that's in that day - muesli, banana, bread, potato. And there's quite a bit of sugar from fruit, too - blueberries, orange juice, banana, kiwifruit and fruit salad.

Breakfast delivers 767 calories and nearly 70 g of sugars (some of this is lactose). Lunch is around 700 calories and 24 g of sugar (mostly from the kiwifruit). Dinner is 508 calories and just a trace of sugars. Snacks add another 591 calories and 58 g of sugar. For the day, then, we have 2566 calories and 152 g of sugars. Most of this sugar is not 'added sugar', so wouldn't be counted under sugar intake recommendations – but it still contributes to your daily intake.

UNCONVENTIONAL HEALTHY
Breakfast:
2 poached eggs, grilled bacon (3 rashers), 1 grilled tomato, ½ an avocado, steamed spinach (½ cup)
Morning tea:
None needed
Lunch:
Large salad with quinoa (½ cup before cooking), mixed vegetables like beetroot, celery, capsicum, cucumber, tomato and snowpeas (2 cups), small can of tuna (95 g), herbs, and a dressing of olive oil (1 tablespoon) and balsamic vinegar or lemon juice (1 tablespoon)
Afternoon tea:
10 almonds
Dinner:
Steak (186 g), peas (50 g), broccoli (100 g), carrots (75 g), sweetcorn (75 g)
Dessert:
Dark chocolate (10 g), peanut butter (1 teaspoon)

Breakfast delivers 777 calories but hardly any sugar, which means that your insulin levels are going to stay steady throughout the morning and you're not going to get the munchies at morning tea time. Lunch is roughly 555 calories, depending on what vegetables you choose to use – this will also affect the sugar content, but let's assume around 10 g of sugar. Dinner comes in at 457 calories with 12.5 g of sugars, mainly from the carrots and sweetcorn. Snacks add up to 156 calories – the sugar content depends on how dark the chocolate is. If you choose 90% cocoa solids, there's virtually no sugar in the chocolate. So for the day we have 1945 calories and 22 g of sugars. That leaves plenty of room for a glass of red, if you fancy it!

So what made the difference? Cutting out some of the white foods like bread and potato, and replacing these with more non-starchy vegetables. Also, removing concentrated sources of sugar like fruit juice. In fact, there's no fruit in this plan. You could add a couple of plums at morning tea and still only add an extra 60 calories – although it would add nearly 14 g of sugars.

#26 EAT A BEAST BREAKFAST

If there's one breakfast that ticks all the nutritional boxes, it's the BEAST – that's Bacon, Egg, Avocado, Spinach and Tomato.

Bacon delivers protein, which helps keep you full through until lunch (if you don't like bacon, swap it out for some salmon; if you don't eat meat, swap it for beans, vege sausage or a nut- or tofu-based product). The egg also provides protein, along with a good dose of minerals and vitamins. The avocado provides plenty of healthy fat, and the spinach and tomato tick off two of your rainbow requirements, delivering a good dose of phytonutrients at the same time. You'll notice that there's no toast – you just don't need it with this meal.

Now, you're not going to eat this for breakfast every day; maybe you'll have it on a Sunday morning, when you've got the time to sit down and enjoy it. But that doesn't mean that breakfast for the rest of the week needs to be a bowl of processed cereal or a couple of slices of toast and jam.

The next few pages contain some other ideas for breakfasts that will be filling and nutritious, and that will set you up for a great day.

BREAKFAST RECIPES

MAKE AHEAD

HOMEMADE NUTTY MUESLI

2 cups oats – preferably wholegrain and large, not flaked into small pieces
½ cup sliced almonds
½ cup raw cashew nuts, chopped
½ cup raw brazil nuts, chopped
½ cup pumpkin seeds
¼ cup chia seeds
1 cup coconut chips (not desiccated coconut)
4 tablespoons coconut oil, melted
4 teaspoons ground cinnamon

Heat the oven to 180°C. Line a large baking tray with greaseproof or baking paper.

Put all of the ingredients in a large bowl and mix well. Spread the mixture out over the baking tray and put it in the oven. Bake for 20 minutes, or until your muesli is lightly toasted. Tip it out onto a large plate to let it cool, then store it in an airtight container.

For breakfast, measure out ½ cup of muesli and add either plain, unsweetened yoghurt or trim milk, plus either a small handful of blueberries or half a banana, chopped.

Supermarket substitute: Don't want to make your own muesli? If you're going to buy a commercial product, check the labels carefully. Look for one that hasn't been sweetened or toasted and check the sugar content – you want one that has less than 20 g per 100 g of muesli (25 g if the muesli contains dried fruit). Try to avoid cereals that have added sweeteners like cane sugar, brown sugar, honey, etc.

OVERNIGHT OATS

This takes 2 minutes to put together in the evening and can be made several days in advance. Uncooked oats are digested more slowly than their cooked counterparts, so will keep you feeling full for longer. You can change up the flavourings and fruit as you like, but you'll get the best nutritional bang from highly coloured fruits like blueberries.

½ cup wholegrain oats
½ cup milk of your choice (unsweetened)
a blob of plain, unsweetened Greek yoghurt
¼ teaspoon ground turmeric
¼ teaspoon ground cinnamon
½ small piece of crystallised ginger, chopped finely (or even better, use fresh ginger)
pinch of salt
½ cup frozen blueberries or other fruit

Combine everything in the dish that you're going to eat out of in the morning. Stir it well, cover with cling film and put in the fridge overnight. In the morning, take it out and eat it! Makes one serving.

CHIA PUDDING

4 tablespoons chia seeds
¾ cup unsweetened almond milk
2 teaspoons ground cinnamon
1 teaspoon vanilla essence or extract
1 teaspoon honey (optional)

To serve
2 tablespoons plain, unsweetened yoghurt
small handful of blueberries or ½ banana, chopped
sprinkle of coconut chips

Place the chia seeds, almond milk, cinnamon, vanilla and honey (if using) in a jar and mix well. Leave to sit for 10 minutes, then mix well again. Cover and put in the fridge overnight. In the morning, add the yoghurt, fruit and coconut chips and eat. Makes one serving.

HOT BREAKFAST

CINNAMON OATS

⅓ cup rolled oats
⅔ cup water, trim milk or unsweetened almond milk
2 teaspoons ground cinnamon
¼ cup shredded coconut
2 tablespoons plain, unsweetened yoghurt
¼ cup blueberries

Place the oats and water or milk in a small saucepan and stir over a medium heat until the mixture has thickened into a porridge (about 10 minutes). Add the cinnamon, then place in a bowl and top with the coconut, yoghurt and blueberries. Makes one serving.

MEDITERRANEAN EGG SCRAMBLE

2 eggs
splash of milk or cream (optional)
butter for cooking
¼ cup green olives
6–8 cherry tomatoes
¼ red onion, finely sliced
1 slice of toast, preferably wholegrain (optional)
handful of rocket leaves

Whisk the eggs, together with the milk or cream if using. Season with salt and pepper.

Melt a small knob of butter in a saucepan, then add the eggs and cook, stirring gently but constantly, so that the eggs scramble. Keep the heat low and remove the pan from the heat just before the eggs look dry – the residual heat in the pan will finish cooking them. Stir through the olives, tomatoes and onion, then pile onto the toast and sprinkle with the rocket. Makes one serving.

Tip: To make great scrambled eggs, cook them for 30 seconds on the heat, then 30 seconds off, then back on and back off again, probably twice more – so 3 minutes in total. Keep stirring, gently, all the time. The eggs will stay soft and moist, with no need to add any liquid.

DRINK IT

GREEN SMOOTHIE

200 ml water or coconut water

1 banana

½ avocado

handful of spinach leaves

⅓ cup plain, unsweetened yoghurt

Blitz all ingredients in a blender, then drink. Makes one serving.

BANANA BERRY SMOOTHIE

200 ml unsweetened almond milk

⅓ cup frozen blueberries

½ medium-sized banana

⅓ cup plain, unsweetened yoghurt

Blitz all ingredients in a blender, then drink. Makes one serving.

BANANA BREAKFAST SMOOTHIE

1 medium-sized banana

⅓ cup rolled oats

100 ml trim milk

100 ml water

⅓ cup plain, unsweetened yoghurt

Blitz all ingredients in a blender, then drink. Makes one serving.

THE LAST RESORT

TOAST WITH BENEFITS

Use wholemeal bread and add toppings with nutritional value.

Suggested toppings:

Avocado and tomato – add fresh basil for a Mediterranean feel

Natural Peanut butter and sliced banana

Hummus – bought if you like or see page 204

Sardines – give yourself an omega-3 boost in the morning

Poached eggs

DON'T SKIP BREAKFAST!

Yes, mornings can be a rush – especially if you have children and a full-time job. But if you want to be healthy, you're going to want to work out a way of fitting breakfast in to your morning routine.

A ground-breaking study has shown that eating breakfast changes the way your body behaves for the rest of the day. Your body has an 'internal clock' which is involved in starting and stopping a wide range of metabolic functions. When you eat breakfast, this clock works in a way that promotes better control of blood sugar and insulin levels. The study showed that people who ate breakfast had better blood sugar control after lunch, compared with days when they didn't eat breakfast.

These results show how skipping breakfast is likely to lead to weight gain, even if you don't eat more later in the day to compensate for the missed meal. The study was conducted with both healthy, normal-weight people and those with diabetes and obesity, with the same outcome for both groups.

So important is the body-clock function that the researchers suggest that proper meal timing could improve overall metabolism, help with weight loss and protect against type 2 diabetes.

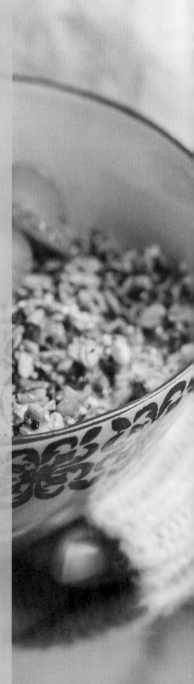

PROGRESS, NOT PERFECTION

Brian, 49

A few years ago I was unfit and overweight, and one day at work I suddenly thought 'What would happen if I couldn't work any more on medical grounds?' It was just a brief thought, but it didn't go away - it just kept nagging at me. But I didn't really do anything about it. Then, in 2014, I got the chance to take part in Nic's programme – and that was the start of a whole new me.

I liked the simplicity of the approach. I didn't need to do a radical overhaul of how I lived - I just needed to make some small adjustments. I'd been doing a bit of exercise - three or four times a week – so I increased that to six or seven times a week, and did a lot more walking.

The big benefit for me came from using MyFitnessPal, which let me see where all my calories were coming from. I remember having a steak dinner at a restaurant and seeing that it came to nearly 1000 calories! The next time I went, I chose the tuna steak and the meal came in at less than half the calories. I used to like a drink, too, but I was getting bothered by my use of alcohol and eventually decided that the best thing for me would be to not drink at all. Through that process I discovered that you only have to not drink one day at a time, and I use this philosophy with my eating and exercise, too. Each day I try to do my best to exercise and make good choices about my food - but if it doesn't work out, I don't dwell on it. I just start again.

I've used Nic's suggestions of experimenting, too. One year it was focusing on addressing my alcohol use, then next it was structured walking sessions with a buddy, and the following year I tried intermittent fasting – and lost 5-6 kg in just a few weeks. Using online shopping helps, too, because you're not tempted by goodies at the supermarket.

I'm so much fitter these days - I've lost a lot of abdominal fat and I don't get so puffed walking up steep hills. It's nice when people say I'm looking trimmer!

The main piece of advice that I'd give someone looking to adopt a more healthy lifestyle is to just take it one day at a time - forever.

#27 LOVE YOUR LUNCH, DIG YOUR DINNER

Even though breakfast is often regarded as the most important meal of the day, for many people lunch and dinner are bigger meals. However, all too often lunch is a sandwich or sushi or a piece of pizza bread from the supermarket – mainly white food with maybe just a smattering of colour. Dinner might be better, with a few more vegetables, but in a lot of homes the main component of an evening meal would be potato, rice or pasta.

Now, there's nothing wrong with these foods if you've got room in your diet for them. If you've expended a lot of energy and you've already eaten all of the veges and good fats and high-quality protein that your body needs, then eating some carbs is going to be fine. But if you've sat on your backside all day and haven't eaten enough vegetables, etc., then – if you want to stay healthy – white food should take a back seat.

HOW TO HAVE A HEALTHY LUNCH

Lunch is often a problem because people aren't organised during the week. As a result, they end up buying lunch or taking a couple of slices of bread to work and slapping together a quick sandwich with a bit of ham or cheese. Or they fall back on convenience foods like noodles or packet soups.

So, how do you avoid this? You get organised.

\# **Plan ahead:** spend a half an hour each week planning what you are going to eat that week. For most people it's the work week that's tough, so focus on this. You know you've got five lunches and five dinners to deal with. Think about what you're going to have, then make sure

BUILD A MEAL

Want to experiment instead of using a recipe? This is pretty easy to do if you're making a main meal or a lunch, but not so easy if you're baking – quantities and ratios are really important for baked goods! If you're going freeform with your cooking, follow these guidelines to help get the best results:

Pick your protein: Choose a protein base for your meal. Some ideas are red meat, chicken, fish, seafood, tofu, tempeh, beans, nuts, cheese, eggs.

Add vegetables: Be sure to include ones that grow above the ground, and make sure you have a mix of colours.

Add texture: If you can get a combination of soft and crunchy in the same mouthful, you've got a much more interesting meal. Raw veg, toasted seeds or nuts, a few croutons – all of these add crunch.

Add flavours: Sometimes a single flavour is OK, but for real interest you'll usually need layers of flavour. A dressing made with a good oil, an acid (e.g. citrus juice or vinegar), a tiny bit of sweet (honey, maple syrup) and maybe a bit of heat (chilli, mustard) will really make a dish pop – with very little effort.

Season your meal: Salt and pepper are the secret ingredients in so many professional kitchens. Make sure you use them when you're cooking – don't leave it until the food is on your plate!

you get what you need to make those meals. Use a meal-planning app, stick a plan up on the fridge, or write it on a chalkboard in your kitchen – whatever works for you.

\# **Prep ahead:** With your plan in place, do as much preparation as possible before the chaos of your work week begins. An hour or two on Sunday spent chopping or cooking can make a phenomenal difference to your diet during the week – and to your stress levels. If you've got kids, see whether you can make this an activity that everyone can help with – it's great for kids to be involved and to learn how to cook.

\# **Make extra:** Leftovers make great lunches! Cook a bit more than you need for dinner, portion it into containers and stick it in the fridge. Or cook extra and freeze it, so that you've got a quick option when your day or week has started to unravel.

\# **Mix 'n' match:** If you've got a stash of vegetables prepared and stored in the fridge, then one day have them with some tinned fish, and the next day have them with some chicken – or whatever protein source takes your fancy. A lot of people find that swapping out the protein introduces enough variety to keep them happy. Consider all of your options – fish, chicken, leftover meat, beans, tofu, egg, cheese, etc.

HOW TO HAVE A HEALTHY DINNER

Being organised is also going to help when it comes to dinner. Instead of getting home and succumbing to the post-work blues by opening a bottle of wine and a packet of chocolate biscuits, or thinking 'I'm hungry, the kids are hungry, everyone's hungry – let's just get takeaways', make sure that you have a plan so that you know what's for dinner each night during the week.

As for lunches, if you've done some preparation on the weekend, then you can get a meal on the table without too much drama during the week. Make good use of 'convenience' foods like frozen vegetables – they can be steamed or microwaved, and are just as nutritious as fresh veg (sometimes even better).

If you have a pressure cooker, use it to produce meals in a fraction of the time that they'd take in the oven or on a stove – with the added benefit that you'll also use less power. Pressure cookers (in particular one called the Instant Pot) are having a bit of a renaissance at the moment, and there are loads of recipe ideas on the internet. Find ones that appeal to you, and give them a go.

The flip-side to a pressure cooker is a slow-cooker. Perfect for winter meals, the slow-cooker can be loaded up in the morning and left all day, so that when you come home all you have to do is dish up.

LEARN HOW TO COOK!

If you don't cook already, have a go. You don't have to make gourmet meals – you just have to make something that is tasty and nutritious. You can start by following recipes. Once you're confident, you can change things up depending on what you have in the cupboard or fridge.

Some good sites for recipes are:

bbcgoodfood.com – has a huge range of recipes for all types of meals. Create a free account and save recipes that you like. They have an app, too.

101cookbooks.com – a big selection of vegetarian recipes, most of which can be changed up quite easily. Has a big focus on natural, unprocessed foods and is easy to search by ingredient.

ohsheglows.com – a great site if you have difficulties with dairy, gluten or other foods. Contains exclusively vegan recipes.

bestrecipes.com.au – has over 15,000 recipes, mostly submitted by users. Nicely organised into different categories to make finding easy recipes easy!

foodlovers.co.nz – family-oriented recipes with a strong focus on fresh, seasonal food. Also has an active forum where you can ask questions.

PIMP YOUR VEGES

So many people say they don't eat veges because they're boring. It's hard to think how this could be true, given that there's such a massive range available. However, if you *do* think that veges are just a bit too dull to eat, here are some simple ways to jazz them up so that you'll want to eat them at every meal.

Salt with sass: Instead of using straight table salt, try getting a few different-flavoured salts and sprinkling these on your veges, especially steamed ones. Try to find salts that have got multiple flavours in them – so chilli-lime salt rather than just lemon salt – as these will add more interest. Don't smother your vegetables with salt, though, as too much salt in your diet increases your risk for high blood pressure. You only need a sprinkle.

Spice it up: Do something different with leafy veges like silverbeet, spinach, kale and cabbage. Put a splash of oil in a frying pan, then gently fry 1 diced onion (red or white) until soft. Add a clove or two of garlic, finely sliced. And if you've got one on hand, add a chilli too (also finely sliced). Cook for a minute, then add some spices – a bit of ginger, some ground turmeric, ground coriander, ground cumin, even just some curry powder if that's what you've got in the cupboard. Make the total amount of spice you add about 2 teaspoons max. Stir the spices through and cook for a minute, then add your leafy veges (which you have washed and cut into strips) and a splash of water. Stir everything through, and cook to your desired level of crispness. Taste to check the seasoning, and add salt if needed.

Slow-braise your veges:
This works well for carrots, celery, cabbage and fennel, and could be adapted for a whole range of veges. Peel your veg, if needed, and cut into bite-sized pieces. Put a knob of butter into a pot that has a well-fitting lid and add a splash of water (about a tablespoon, maybe two). Put the veg in, add salt and pepper (freshly ground tastes so much better), give it a stir, put the lid on and put the pot on the stove on a medium heat. As soon as you hear the water start to bubble and hiss, turn the heat down to the lowest setting and leave for 20–30 minutes. Check it once or twice during the cooking time – give it a stir and add a small splash of water if it looks like it's going to burn.

Drizzle them with flavoured oils:
This works really well on steamed veges, like broccoli. Buy a small bottle of a nice flavoured oil – lemon-flavoured avocado oil, for example – and put a light drizzle of this over the veges on your plate. You probably won't even need to add any salt.

Add crunch:
Virtually any vegetable can be pepped up with a crunchy topping sprinkled over the top, but steamed or boiled veges particularly benefit from this. Sprinkle the cooked veg with some dukkah (buy it or make your own – it's easy and keeps for ages), or some spiced seeds (see the recipe on page 205), or even some garlic-infused crunchy breadcrumbs – blitz a slice or two of stale bread in a food processor (or crumble by hand), heat a mix of butter and olive oil in a frying pan, add a few sliced cloves of garlic, some finely chopped chilli and a couple of anchovies, then toss in the breadcrumbs and cook till they brown up. They'll go crispy as they cool.

#28 SNACK SMART

Snack attack! We've all been there. Whether it's mid-morning and you haven't had enough breakfast, mid-afternoon and you're bored at work or stressed with the kids, or after-dinner couch time and you just feel like something else to reward yourself for getting through the day – cravings can hit at any time.

Snacks are an integral part of modern life. In fact, some people don't bother with sit-down meals and just snack all day! All too often, though, the snacks we eat are high in sugar, high in salt and/or high in saturated fat. They make you feel good – temporarily – but they undo a healthy diet and leave you worse off in the long run.

The good news is that snacking can be part of a healthy lifestyle. It all comes down to what you snack on.

BAD WAYS OF SNACKING

If you want to get the most out of your snacks, try to avoid the following:

Foods that are high in sugar: Biscuits, cakes, chocolates, sweets, a lot of commercial muesli bars.

Foods that are mainly white carbs: Biscuits, cakes, a lot of commercial muesli bars, sandwiches, potato chips.

Foods that are high in fat: Potato chips, chocolate, sausage rolls, meat pies.

Foods that are processed: Biscuits, cakes – you get the picture . . .

GOOD WAYS OF SNACKING

So now that all the easily available items have been removed from the snack equation, what's left?

1. First, figure out whether you're actually hungry. Are you just bored or stressed instead? If yes, is there something else you can do to change how you feel?

2. Second, check that you're not thirsty. We often eat when really we need to drink. Even if you think you're not thirsty, have a drink anyway – sometimes this takes away the urge to snack.

3. Next, consider whether you included enough protein in your last meal. Protein tends to keep us feeling fuller for longer, reducing the need to snack. Of course, you can't go back in time and have your breakfast again, but you can make a note to adjust the protein content for the next time.

4. Now, opt for snacks that deliver both nutrients and fibre. You're mostly not going to find these in a vending machine at work, or even in the corner store, so you're going to have to be prepared.

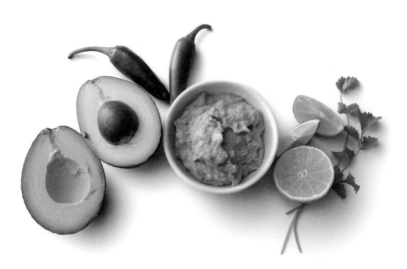

SOME GREAT SNACK RECIPES

Here are some great ideas for things to take to work, on the road, or just as far as the couch!

MAKE AHEAD

HUMMUS

400 g can chickpeas
1 clove garlic, crushed
1 lemon, zest and juice
3 tablespoons tahini
pinch of ground cumin
good-quality olive oil

Tip the chickpeas into a sieve, rinse with cold water and drain. Put them in a food processor together with the garlic, lemon zest and juice, tahini and cumin, and whizz it all up to a paste. Add a splash of water to get the consistency you want – it should look lovely and creamy – and adjust the flavour to your taste using more garlic, lemon and/or tahini. Put the hummus in a container and drizzle with a bit of olive oil. Store in an airtight container in the fridge – it should keep for a week.

No food processor? Mash everything together in a bowl with a fork or a potato masher – you'll get a bonus upper body workout as well as your hummus!

Don't want to make your own? Buy a good-quality ready-made version from the supermarket (check the labels).

Serve with peeled carrots cut into sticks and/or celery stalks cut into manageable pieces. (Too busy? Buy baby carrots and pre-cut celery at the supermarket.) If you're taking this into work, invest in some small clip-lid plastic containers so that you've got portion control. A single snack portion of hummus is about ¼ cup.

GUACAMOLE

1 tomato
2 avocados
juice of 1 small lime
1 clove garlic, crushed
¼ red onion, finely diced
fresh chilli and/or fresh coriander (optional)

Dice the tomato finely, put it in a sieve and leave it over a bowl or the sink to drain. Meanwhile, peel the avocados and mash the flesh together with the lime juice. Stir through the garlic and red onion, along with the finely diced chilli and/or chopped fresh coriander, if using. Finally, stir through the diced, drained tomato. Taste, and add salt if needed. Store in an airtight container in the fridge and use within a couple of days.
Don't want to make your own? Buy some ready-made guacamole from the supermarket. It won't taste as good as home-made, but it's easy if you're in a hurry.

Serve with carrot sticks and/or celery stalks. (Too busy? Buy baby carrots and pre-cut celery at the supermarket.) If you're taking this into work, invest in some small plastic containers so that you've got portion control. A single snack portion of guacamole is about ¼ cup.

SPICED SEEDS

250 g mixed seeds – pumpkin and sunflower are best
1 teaspoon spice of your choice – garam masala or ras el hanout are good options
1 teaspoon sweetener – maple syrup, agave syrup, rice bran syrup (not honey – it will make everything too sticky)
1 teaspoon tamari, soy sauce or other liquid to complement your spice
1 teaspoon vegetable oil
½ teaspoon flaky salt
pinch of chilli or cayenne, if you want a bit of heat

Preheat the oven to 160°C.
Mix all the ingredients together in a bowl, then tip onto a baking tray and spread out evenly. Cook for 15–20 minutes, being careful not to let the seeds burn. Loosen any stuck seeds from the tray, and tip out onto a large plate to cool. Store in an airtight container at room temperature.

SPICY POPCORN

½ cup popcorn kernels
2 tablespoons coconut oil
2 tablespoons maple syrup or equivalent sweetener (not honey)
½ teaspoon chilli powder
½ teaspoon ground cumin
½ teaspoon ground turmeric
½ teaspoon flaky salt

Preheat the oven to 175°C. Pop the popcorn in an air popper (if you don't have an air popper, follow the instructions on the popcorn package).

Place the coconut oil on a large baking tray and put it in the oven until it's just melted. Remove the tray, then stir the maple syrup, spices and salt into the coconut oil.

Tip in the popped popcorn, and stir with your hands to coat all of the popcorn with the mixture. Remove any unpopped kernels as you go, or you'll end up with a mess all over your oven!

Spread the popcorn out evenly over the tray, put it in the oven and bake for about 8 minutes. Remove and let it cool slightly. Store in an airtight container at room temperature.

MIX AND MATCH

CRACKERS AND TOPPINGS

Pick a cracker variety that has a good wholegrain content, is relatively low in saturated fat and doesn't have loads of sugar or salt. Check the label to see how many calories per cracker – your snack portion is about 100 calories, so that's four 25-calorie crackers or two 50-calorie crackers. Choose wisely!

Top with any of the following:
A slice of avocado, a slice of tomato, salt and pepper
Marmite (no butter) and a slice of tomato
Hummus
Guacamole
A smear of peanut butter and a couple of slices of banana
A big slice of tomato, salt and pepper and a few fresh basil leaves

EASY

NUTS

Buy raw, unsalted nuts from the supermarket or your preferred food store. Portion them out into servings of 10-12 nuts (4-5 if they are Brazil nuts).

APPLE AND PEANUT BUTTER

Slice an apple in half and use a spoon to scoop out the core.
Put ½ teaspoon of peanut butter into the cavity of each apple half.

CARROT, CELERY AND PEANUT BUTTER

Cut carrots and celery into sticks and smear them with a bit of peanut butter.

SNACK IN A CAN

Open a small can of tuna or salmon! Choose cans that provide around 100 calories (420 kilojoules) per serving. There are some great flavours available, but watch out for added sugar.

BLISS BALLS

NUT AND OAT BLISS BALLS

1 cup rolled oats
½ cup peanut butter or almond butter
½ cup dates, diced
1 tablespoon coconut oil
1 tablespoon chia seeds
2 tablespoons cacao nibs or cocoa powder (optional)
1 tablespoon pumpkin seeds
1 teaspoon ground cinnamon
pinch of salt
handful of desiccated coconut, for coating
Blitz all of the ingredients except the desiccated coconut in a food processor, until they come together into a firm paste. Form tablespoons of the mixture into balls, then roll in desiccated coconut. Freeze.
Either eat frozen, or take a couple out to take to work.

SUPER-SALADS

Having a stash of salads in the fridge is one of the easiest ways to add vegetables to your meals. Salad can be made with raw or cooked vegetables, whichever takes your fancy. Raw salads are great in summer because they're so fresh and cooling, and they're pretty easy to roll out if you're having a barbecue in the evening. There are heaps of ideas for salads on the internet, but here are a few to get you started.

\# **Beetroot and carrot:** Peel the beetroot, but you can just scrub the carrots if you like. Grate equal amounts of beetroot and carrot. Put them in a bowl and add a handful of sultanas and a big handful each of finely chopped mint and parsley leaves. Put a good handful of pumpkin seeds into a dry frying pan and toast them until they just start to colour; tip them into a bowl to cool, then do the same to a handful of sunflower seeds. While the toasted seeds are cooling, make a dressing. Whisk together 2 tablespoons each of olive oil and orange juice, 1 tablespoon each of pomegranate molasses and balsamic vinegar, and add a touch of honey if you want more sweetness. Pour this over the salad mix, add the seeds and stir everything so that it's all mixed together. (Don't have pomegranate molasses? Substitute maple syrup or a bit more honey.)

\# **Green goodness:** Cook 200 g frozen edamame beans in the microwave, drain and leave to cool; do the same with 200 g frozen peas. Finely chop a small bunch of spring onions, including the green parts, and put them in a bowl. Cut an avocado (or two) into nice bite-sized pieces and add to the bowl along with the juice of 1 lemon, 1 teaspoon of ground cumin and some salt to taste. Finely shred a big handful of flat-leaf parsley and a big handful of mint leaves; add some chopped chives, too, if you like. Add this to bowl, along with some diced cucumber (the little Lebanese ones are nice). Add the cooked peas and beans, and mix to combine.

- # **Brassica bowl 1:** Cut a large head of broccoli (or two smaller heads) into bite-sized florets. Bring a big pot of water to the boil, add salt, then toss in the broccoli for 1–2 minutes – you're just taking the raw edge off them, not cooking them. Tip them into a colander straight away, then rinse them in ice-cold water to stop the cooking process (it will also help keep them nice and green). Grate a couple of carrots into a bowl, and add the broccoli. Make a dressing by combining equal quantities of olive oil and fresh lemon juice (a tablespoon of each will be plenty), with some chilli flakes (or fresh chilli, if you like), salt and pepper. Stir through the vegetables.

- # **Brassica bowl 2:** Cut a medium-sized cauliflower into bite-sized florets. Bring a big pot of water to the boil, add salt, then toss in the cauliflower for 1–2 minutes only. Drain in a colander and rinse with ice-cold water to stop the cooking process. Make sure the cauliflower drains well – you might even want to pat it dry with a paper towel – then put it in a bowl. Add a big bunch of finely sliced flat-leaf parsley. Halve some pitted black olives and add those. If you have capers (the ones preserved in salt), rinse some and add them as well. If you want extra crunch and colour, add a finely diced red capsicum. Make a dressing by combining equal quantities of olive oil and red wine vinegar (a tablespoon of each will be plenty), then stir this through the salad, adding salt and pepper if desired.

- # **Tomato salad:** Take some firm, fresh tomatoes and either slice them or cut them into segments. If you've got cherry tomatoes, just halve them. Finely shred a good handful of mint leaves and put this into a bowl with the tomatoes. If you want a bit of zing, add some finely sliced spring onion or shallot. Make a dressing with equal amounts of olive oil and fresh lemon juice (a tablespoon of each should be enough), plus salt and pepper. Gently stir the dressing through. This tastes better if left for half an hour or so for the flavours to develop.

#29 BUT I'M EATING OUT

Eating out is part of everyday life for a lot of people. While it's fun, it can be a minefield if you're trying to eat healthily. One reason? White food.

When it comes to catering, you're going to see a lot of white food. In a café? Look at the cakes, muffins, biscuits, pies, pastries, sandwiches, rolls, wraps, baps – virtually everything on offer will have a decent amount of flour in it somewhere. And it doesn't matter whether it's gluten-free or not – we're still talking finely milled grains that will send your blood insulin spiralling and spike your blood glucose before you can finish your coffee!

What about sushi? Most people think that's a nice, healthy meal. But look at all that white rice – if all you have is a few pieces of sushi, then you're going to be hungry again in next to no time. Your blood sugars will rise quickly and fall just as fast, leaving you craving something sweet to fill the gap.

How about the classic fast-food items – burgers, fried chicken, pizza, and fish and chips? Burgers come with buns, and normally there's a decent side of fries, too. That's two servings of white food right there. Add a drink and you've got a third, thanks to the sugar. Fried chicken normally comes with something white, too - fries or mashed potato or garlic bread – oh, and a drink, of course. Pizza – well, that's obviously just bread with toppings. And while the fish in fish and chips might be good for you, the batter's flour-based and those chips were definitely a potato before they were cooked.

HOW TO EAT OUT YOUR WAY

There's a reason why white food dominates these types of meal – it's cheap, it's easy and we love it. But, as the paying customer, you have the power to choose what you eat.

The simplest option is not to eat out – but that's not going to work all the time. When you do eat out, then, make a conscious effort to choose items that are low in white foods. Cafés often have good salad selections nowadays, and they're usually happy to do a half-and-half mix, so you can get two different ones on the one plate. Choose this and be the envy of your mates, sitting there with their paninis.

If the café doesn't have anything on the menu that appeals, you've got a few choices. You can suck it up and just get something that will do the least damage to your health efforts (a good option if you're with friends), you can walk out and try a different place, or you can ask the staff whether the kitchen can prepare something slightly off-menu. As long as you're pleasant about it and don't demand something completely outrageous, cafés are usually happy to adapt an existing item for customers. If you were having Eggs Benedict, say, you could ask for just a single slice of toast or half the bagel, instead of the full item. That reduces waste, and also reduces the risk that you're going to eat everything just out of habit.

If you're going out for dinner, you've got similar options. Evening meals in restaurants often aren't that carb-heavy, as you're paying more for what you're getting. Opt for dishes that feature a lean protein, and add in extra veg or salad. If the dish usually comes with rice or pasta or potatoes on the side, just ask if they can be left off.

Of course, sometimes it's just not that easy. You might have restricted dining options – maybe the work canteen is your only choice, and they excel at stodge. If you're in this situation occasionally, then just relax and go with the flow. But if it's every day, then you need to find an alternative strategy that lets you stay in control of your health. Taking the time the night before to pack a lunch for the next day (and even for the day after that, if you can) will make all the difference. It doesn't have to be complicated, either – take a look at some of the suggestions on page 187 and pages 196-7.

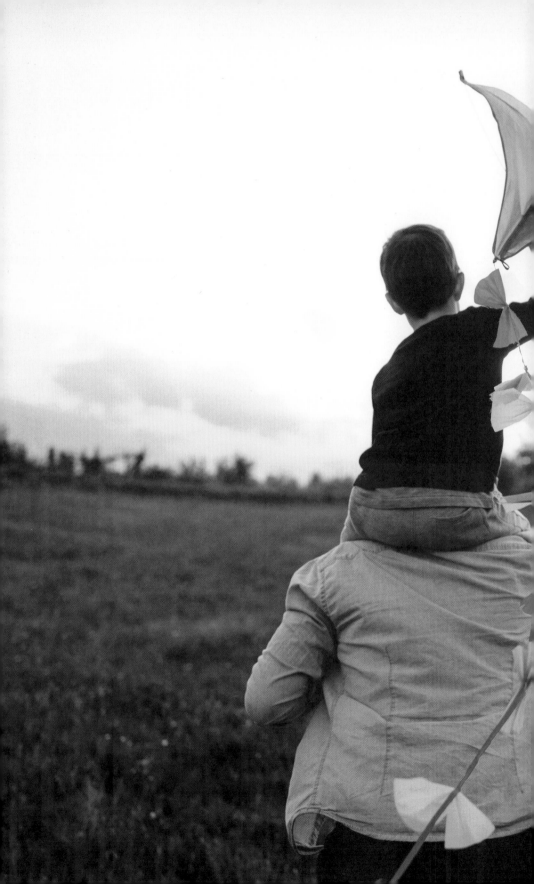

PART FIVE

—

NOW, WHAT ARE YOU GOING TO DO?

If you've made it this far, you should have all of the information you need to be your own health guru. You'll have a good idea of how your body works, and how different types of activity can help maintain it in good condition. You'll understand what foods deliver real value for your health and how to get more of these foods on your plate each day. Importantly, you'll have a good idea of what you want to change in your life, and what factors might help or hinder you. Now, it's time to put it all together, to build a plan that works for you. This might be a structured plan that details your food and exercise for every day, or a flexible plan that contains guidelines you can adapt if circumstances change. Or it might just be a list of tweaks that you want to make to gradually transform your life. Regardless of what approach you choose, the first step is taking a look at what makes you tick.

#30 WHAT MAKES YOU TICK?

What makes you happy? Specifically, what makes you happy when it comes to health and food and fitness? Is it having a routine that means you don't have to make decisions each day? Is it novelty? Is it freedom, or flexibility? Does setting a goal and working towards it make you smile, or is it achieving it that's the fun part? Do you feel happier doing something good for yourself, or for others?

On the flip side, what makes you unhappy? A lack of control; deprivation; feeling like a failure; feeling hemmed in by other people's expectations; a sense that you're drifting through life; feeling left out. All of these things can make people feel down. Does the idea of a challenge like tackling your health just feel too hard?

START FIGURING IT OUT

If you keep a journal – paper or digital – go grab it now. If not, grab a bit of paper or open up a note app on your phone or tablet.

Now, spend some time thinking about your triggers for happiness, and about the things that make you unhappy. Write them down. You don't have to show them to anyone else, but you do need to see them yourself. Just thinking about them won't make them real enough. This might be quite a difficult exercise, especially if you've never thought about this type of thing before. You might need a few attempts to discover exactly what it is that affects your happiness.

Once you've done that, think about how you behave when you want to achieve something. What drives you to do things? What's your motivation? We're all different, so there is no single 'right' answer to this question. Some of us are motivated by

WHAT ARE MY TRIGGERS?

We've all got our triggers and traits that trip us up – unless we're aware of them. I know that I have an addictive personality and that means that I take an all-or-nothing approach to life! But because I know this, I can watch out for it affecting my health.

Before I realised this, I'd train like crazy and then I'd eat like crazy to make up for all the energy I was burning. The trouble with this approach was that I didn't get the full benefit of the exercise I was doing – all I got was fatigue and illness. I had to learn to moderate my exercise and to eat to support my body, so that it could get stronger rather than just recovering from the exercise.

money, some by power, some by knowledge. Some of us are motivated by pleasure, others by avoiding pain. Some people want to be seen as the best and others want to be able to help people.

How can you harness the way you're motivated to help yourself? Say you're motivated by avoiding pain. If you're 35 now, and you're not terribly healthy, you might not be feeling the effects – yet. But imagine what you'll be like in another 10 or 20 years. Think about older family members who might fall into this category – are they suffering because they're not healthy? Sit in a shopping mall or at a café, and watch people for a while – how many of them are moving slowly or awkwardly and are clearly not in good health? Can you see yourself ending up like this? Can you use that as motivation to make a change?

TAKE A CLOSE LOOK AT YOURSELF

Now, think about your personal characteristics that might get in the way of your success. Maybe you've got an addictive personality. Maybe you've got a tendency to be a bit lazy. Maybe you're a perfectionist. Be honest with yourself when you're identifying these traits. If you can't think of anything, ask a family member or friend who you can trust to give you some honest insight. It's often easier to see others more clearly than we can see ourselves.

Once you've identified these traits, consider how you can manage them so they don't stop you achieving your goals. Maybe you can even turn them to your advantage. Say you know you get addicted to things – you just *have* to eat chocolate every day, or you *have* to binge-watch an entire series on TV, or when you open a bottle of wine you can't rest until it's finished. Can you consciously turn this attribute into something more positive? Can you tell yourself that you're going to get addicted to eating a healthy meal every lunchtime, because you like the admiring comments you'll get from others? Or maybe that you're going to get addicted to doing strength training three times a week, because you're going to get a buzz from seeing yourself get stronger? It might take a bit of work to turn a negative into a positive, but it's worth the effort.

WHY DO YOU EAT?

We all eat for many different reasons: out of habit, from boredom, to be sociable, to fill an emotional gap – and sometimes we even eat because we're hungry. If you want to change how you eat, so that you adopt a healthier approach to food, then you need to understand why *you* eat.

Take a moment to look back over the past week. Think about all of the times you ate during that week, and why you ate. Write these down, so that you have a visual record of what you've done – and be honest with yourself. If you ate a half a packet of chocolate biscuits on Sunday evening because the thought of going to work the next day made you feel sad and depressed, then you need to know that. If you only ate a light salad at lunch

217

because you didn't want to look greedy in front of your work colleagues, but then scoffed a chocolate bar in secret later in the afternoon because you were starving, that's OK too – you just need to know it. If you missed meals, then record why you didn't eat them.

SOME REASONS WE DON'T EAT

- # Too busy.
- # Running late.
- # Stuck in a meeting.
- # Stuck in traffic.
- # Not hungry.
- # Not inspired by anything on offer.
- # Couldn't afford it.
- # Saving my appetite for later.
- # Trying to cut back on how much I eat.
- # Didn't want to look greedy.
- # Feel uncomfortable eating with others.
- # Feel uncomfortable eating alone.
- # I don't like the way my body looks.
- # Just forgot.

SOME REASONS WE DO EAT

- # Hungry!
- # Free food is on offer.
- # Social – others are eating.
- # Someone else has cooked for me.
- # It's breakfast/lunch/dinner time.
- # Got a craving for chocolate/chips/alfalfa sprouts.
- # Love the taste of food.
- # Bored!
- # Feeling sad or lonely.
- # Habit – e.g. 'I always eat when I watch TV'.
- # Trying to gain weight.
- # Trying to gain muscle.
- # To fuel my body.
- # I don't like the way my body looks.

WHY DO I EAT?

I'm a real foodie – I love food. But at the same time, I love being fit and healthy – so what I eat needs to tick both of those boxes.

Some of the food I eat is very much geared towards ensuring that I can train hard, so that I can meet my sporting goals. That's where my protein, my vegetables, my healthy fats come in. Once I've met my body's needs with the really good stuff, then I can add other foods that I love – things that aren't necessarily bad for me, but are more like the optional extras on top of the basics. For me, that's dark chocolate, red wine, beer, popcorn, peanut butter and cheese – but not all on the same plate!

I'm a really sociable person and love eating with friends and family. By making good decisions about my day-to-day diet, I can quite happily enjoy those social meals without compromising my health. There are also some foods that I really enjoy eating in certain situations, and there's no way I'll be happy if I can't have them. I absolutely love sausages and beer in summer, so I'll eat really well during the day, throw in a bit of exercise and then, in the evening, I'll have the freedom to eat the things that make me happy.

Now, look at your list and think about which of your eating patterns support your pursuit of a healthy lifestyle. Are there any that you can reduce – or do more frequently – to help you eat in a more healthy way? Are there any that you could, realistically, give up completely? Unless you're going to move to the top of a mountain and live like a hermit, it's not realistic to give up eating for social reasons – a meal with friends and/or family is a great thing, not something to deny yourself. But eating because you're bored doesn't have any particular benefit, so that would be a habit you could look at changing.

WHY DO I EXERCISE?

I love what exercise does for me. Probably the best thing that happens is that I get more out of my day when I'm fit. I'm more productive, I'm happier, I've got more energy, I sleep better.

Yes, exercise makes me physically stronger, but it also makes me mentally stronger – and that flows through to all other parts of my life. When I've taken the time to look after myself, by doing some exercise that invigorates and challenges me, I've got so much more to give to other people – family, friends, work colleagues. It's just a real win-win.

I love the challenge, too – I like to see how far I can push my body and defy my age. I want to see how much better I can get in the sport that I do. The bonus is that I look healthy and I feel healthy. And because I'm burning a fair bit of energy, I get to eat not just the food I need for fuel and function, but also the food I love to eat.

Once you've been through this exercise, write yourself a personal statement that describes the way you want to eat. Keep it reasonably short. An example could be: 'I want to eat in a way that lets me have a strong body, and also lets me enjoy good food and not get hung up about my diet.' Make it personal to you. Write it on a small bit of paper, then put that paper somewhere you can look at it easily. Maybe photograph it and leave it on your phone, or put the paper in your purse or wallet, or stick it in the pocket of your jacket. Then, for the next couple of weeks, read your statement before every meal or snack, to check that what you're about to do is in line with what you *want* to do.

NOW, WHAT ARE YOU GOING TO DO?

What makes you happy?

....

....

....

What makes you unhappy?

....

....

....

What motivates you?

....

....

....

How can you use this motivation?

....

....

....

WHAT DO YOU TELL YOURSELF ABOUT EXERCISE?

As kids, most of us loved to exercise. We ran around, screaming, shouting, laughing – having heaps of fun. But somehow, as we get older, some of us lose this. We start seeing exercise as something negative; as something that's going to intrude on our leisure time. And the more we tell ourselves this, the more we believe it.

EXCUSES FOR WHY SOME OF US DON'T EXERCISE

- I don't enjoy it.
- I'm too busy.
- It's too boring.
- I've got a sore knee/hip/shoulder/elbow.
- It's too expensive.
- I'm no good at it.
- I *just can't* run/swim/bike/do anything other than sit on the couch and eat potato chips.

REASONS WHY SOME OF US LOVE EXERCISE

- It makes me feel alive.
- It helps me get more out of my day.
- I love the challenge.
- I love feeling strong.
- I love seeing myself progressing and improving.
- I love the social side.
- It's important to invest time in me.
- There's so many different options to try.

Get out the notebook or app you used earlier, and write down how you feel about exercise – all the negative things and all the positive things. Just like you did with the eating exercise, be honest with yourself.

Now look at the negative things on your list. Ask yourself if they are really what's stopping you – or are they just excuses? In most cases, you'll find they're excuses. We tell ourselves a story, and create barriers that stop us seeing alternatives. So we say we can't exercise because we can't afford a gym membership. Rubbish. There is no need to join a gym to get exercise. We say we're no good at it – but that's true of anything until we learn how to do it. We tell ourselves it's boring – but that's a cop-out; boredom is just a state of mind.

There's no magic bullet or food or formula for changing your view of exercise. Be honest with yourself, and then challenge yourself. Experiment with different types of exercise, alone or with people, outdoors or indoors, paid or free. Dabble in everything, and find something that makes you happy and makes you feel good. Once you've got that, you can start telling yourself a different, more positive story about how you feel about exercise.

How do you feel about exercise?

....

....

....

....

How could you change any negatives?

....

....

....

....

#31 EXPERIMENT ESSENTIALS

Every one of us is different, which means that the things that will get you a healthy lifestyle are subtly different to the things that will work for your best friend or your neighbour or your favourite celebrity. You can read as many diet or exercise books as you like, binge-watch TV shows about health, or religiously follow someone's advice on Twitter – but there's not much chance that the information you get is going to be ideal for you and your life.

The only way to get a truly personalised approach to your health is to experiment – on yourself. Experiments are easy to do, but to get useful information from them you need to follow some guidelines.

GUIDELINES FOR GOOD EXPERIMENTS

1. Decide what you're going to test, and why and how.
2. Before you change anything, measure your baseline.
3. Make the change – but leave everything else the same.
4. Measure your outcome, and interpret the results objectively.
5. Repeat the experiment.

Let's take a closer look at each of these steps.

STEP 1: DECIDE WHAT YOU'RE GOING TO TEST, AND WHY AND HOW

When you're setting up an experiment, you need to have a clear understanding of what you're investigating. Let's say that you thought broccoli was bad for you and you'd be much better if you didn't eat it.

First, you need to define what you mean by 'broccoli'. Sounds easy – but are you talking about raw broccoli or cooked broccoli? Is it still bad for you if it's in a muffin? Or in blue cheese and broccoli soup? Or in a green smoothie?

Next, you need to be clear about why you're testing this out. What do you think broccoli does to you that's bad for your health? Does it make you burp more? Does it give you indigestion? Do you think it makes you tired? Do you think it makes you put on weight?

Once you've identified the 'why', you can work out how you're going to test this. If you believe that raw broccoli makes you tired, then you don't need to measure how often you burp!

STEP 2: BEFORE YOU CHANGE ANYTHING, MEASURE YOUR BASELINE

When scientists conduct an experiment, they normally have a 'control group' that experiences everything that the test group does except for the one factor that is being tested. Say that we wanted to see the effect of a cupcake with lunch on the attention of 5-year-old children at school. We could take a class of 30 children, all the same age, all boys, all of whom had the same breakfast before they came to school. Then we'd split the group into two, put them into separate but identical lunch rooms, and give them exactly the same meal – except that one group would also get a cupcake. (We keep them separate because we don't want the other group to know that they're missing out on a cupcake; otherwise that could affect their behaviour.) Then we'd bring all the children back into the same classroom and have some observers in the room who would rate the attention of the children, using a scale that had already been tested. Importantly, the observers wouldn't know who had had a cupcake and who hadn't, so that couldn't influence how they judged the children's behaviour.

This sort of experiment is called a controlled, blind experiment, and it's a very good way to get unbiased information about what we're testing. Clearly, though, when we're experimenting on ourselves we can't do this sort of experiment! To overcome this, we have to use ourselves as the control group as well as the test group. That means we need to be honest with ourselves and be objective in our measurements – otherwise we won't see the truth; we'll only see what we want to see.

To use yourself as a control, you need to measure your baseline. That means measuring where you are now, before you start to make the change you want to test. Let's use the example 'I want to test whether raw broccoli makes me tired'. For a week before you start the experiment, you'd need to eat raw broccoli every day and rate how tired you felt, using the same scale that you're going to use in your experiment. An easy way to do this would be to rate your tiredness on a scale of 1 to 10, every hour, and to also record how much sleep you got each night. You'd also need to record what other activities you did that week, so that you had a clear picture of everything that could affect the experiment.

After a week, you'd have a good baseline. Let's say that you found you got an average of 6 hours sleep a night and had an average tiredness score of 8 out of 10.

STEP 3: MAKE THE CHANGE – BUT LEAVE EVERYTHING ELSE THE SAME

Now you'll get right into the heart of the experiment. For the next week, you'll cut out raw broccoli from your diet but you won't change anything else. You'll still eat cooked broccoli, you'll still go to bed at the same time, you'll still spend a full day at work and the evening sorting out the kids and the weekend rushing round doing chores and a bit of socialising. *Phew!* And every day, you'll rate your tiredness on a scale of 1 to 10, every hour, and you'll record how much sleep you got each night.

STEP 4: MEASURE YOUR OUTCOME, AND INTERPRET THE RESULTS OBJECTIVELY

After a week of the experiment, you'll be ready to measure the result. Compare your baseline scores with your experiment scores. If they're both pretty similar, you can conclude that raw broccoli doesn't make you tired – it must be something else. If you see that you were less tired in the week when you didn't eat raw broccoli, but you notice that you got an average of 8 hours sleep, then you'd need to do some more investigation. Did you

TRY THIS

If you think you're the sort of person who *just can't* do something different, then try this challenge. It doesn't take any time out of your day, it doesn't cost you any money and you don't need any special gear.

All you have to do is move the shower control from hot to cold. For five days, try taking a cold shower. It doesn't even have to be the whole shower. Start out warm, then finish with a nice, cold, 20-second blast to wake yourself up. Or, alternate hot and cold to give yourself a real endorphin rush.

You're not going to burn heaps of extra energy, or get glowing skin, or magically heal an old injury by doing this. It's just a mind game. What it will show you is that you are strong and that if you set your mind to it, you *just can* do something different!

get more sleep because you didn't eat raw broccoli, or was there something else that affected your sleep? You'd need to look at your record of activities for the two weeks to get a clue as to what it might be.

STEP 5: REPEAT THE EXPERIMENT

Repeating experiments helps you validate the results, which is especially important when you're the only person in the experiment! Depending on the experiment, you might want to do it three times to really make sure that what you're seeing is true.

If you repeat the raw broccoli experiment and find that this time your baseline sleep (when you were eating raw broccoli) averaged 8 hours and when you eliminated broccoli from your diet you only averaged 6 hours a night, then you'd have a pretty good indication that it wasn't the broccoli that was making you tired!

A LITTLE REVIEW

Once you start doing experiments on yourself, you can find they're a lot of fun. An experiment doesn't have to be complicated or expensive, or even last for very long. You can do experiments that last for a day, a week or a month – or any other length of time that works for you!

Before you jump in and start experimenting, take a few moments to revisit the goals that you set way back at the beginning of this journey (see page 30). Are there any of those goals that you could test out with an experiment or two? If one of your goals was to give up sugar in your tea and coffee, then that would be an easy place to start. If your goals were bigger – say to run a half-marathon – then could you create some smaller goals that would help you get there, and use those for experiments?

Now is also a good time to review your current situation. What's stopping you from changing? What might stop you from changing? How can you address these issues to give yourself the best chance of success? Take a look back at pages 31 to 37 if you've forgotten the common challenges you're likely to face. Before you launch into any experiments, clear the decks of these issues – or at least, have an idea of how you're going to manage them.

ONE-DAY EXPERIMENTS

One-day experiments are a great place to start. They don't involve making huge changes to your lifestyle and they don't need a massive amount of commitment or willpower. Use one-day experiments to see how it feels to stop something that you do habitually, or to test what it might feel like to start something new. Here's a month's worth of one-day experiments:

1. Give up sugar in your tea or coffee – what does it taste like now? Can you detect more flavours or different flavours?
2. If you're a caffeine junkie (tea, coffee, energy drinks), go without for one day. You'll probably feel awful (because it takes a while to wean the body off a caffeine addiction), but at least you'll have proved that you can do it.

3. Replace sugary soda drinks with water for the day – what does this do to your appetite and energy levels?
4. Try a high-protein, high-fat, low-carbohydrate breakfast. What does this do to your sense of hunger later in the day? Do you feel fuller for longer?
5. If you normally skip breakfast, try eating it – how does that affect your energy levels during the day?
6. Swap your morning biscuits or muffin for some nuts – how does that affect how hungry you are at lunchtime?
7. If you always buy lunch, try taking your own to work – does it taste better?
8. If you normally graze all day, try just eating three healthy meals – how does it make you feel?
9. If you normally eat really fast, try eating all your food with chopsticks for one day – see if you still eat as much as you usually would.
10. Try restricting your eating to a set time period, like a 12-hour window (7 am to 7 pm) – does it feel like something you could do more often?
11. Spend a day without eating any white foods (e.g. potatoes, white rice, pasta, white bread, sugar, cakes, biscuits). Did you find you missed them?
12. Eat when you're actually hungry, instead of eating when the clock says you should. Do you think you ate less than normal?
13. Going for the whole day without eating any foods with added sugar. Do you think you could repeat this for another day?
14. Scale back your portion sizes for your meals – try only eating three-quarters of what you normally would. Did you feel hungrier at the end of the day, or not?
15. Go alcohol-free for the day. Was it as difficult as you imagined?
16. Spend a day getting in as much incidental walking as you can – take the stairs, park as far away from buildings as you can, go and talk to your co-workers instead of sending them an email. Could you build this in to your day more regularly?

17. Try doing a 20-minute walk before breakfast. How did you feel for the rest of the day?

18. Get up 30 minutes earlier and do any sort of exercise before breakfast – walk, yoga, stretching, anything that gets your body moving. How did you feel for the rest of the day?

19. Try standing up and walking around whenever you're on the phone. Could you build this up to be a habit?

20. If you're watching TV, do some sort of exercise during the ad breaks. Could you make this a habit?

21. Try getting out for a walk during your lunch break – what does this do for your energy levels in the afternoon?

22. Give your lawn-mowing company the day off and do it yourself – could you make this a regular thing?

23. Swap out a short car journey – walk or cycle instead. Can you do this more regularly?

24. Have screen-free time for an hour before you go to bed – see if you fall asleep more easily.

25. Try going to bed half an hour earlier – do you feel more rested in the morning?

26. Avoid the snooze button. Instead, get up when you wake up or when your alarm goes off – do you have more energy as a result?

27. Download a 'relaxing sounds' app – see if it helps you drift off to sleep more easily.

28. Try meditating or a similar relaxing activity – do you feel calmer, or less stressed?

29. Eat dinner at the table instead of in front of the TV – are you more aware of what you're eating?

30. Spend some time just sitting and watching nature: birds in the garden, trees blowing in the wind, rain sweeping across the street – do these activities help calm and de-stress you?

31. If you can, spend a bit of time in nature: on a beach, in a forest or in a park in the city – how does it affect the rest of your day?

One-day experiments are testing grounds. Sometimes, you'll do a one-day test and find that it was really easy – you'd have no trouble keeping it up for a week. That's a great result – you've proven to yourself that you can do it. Other times, though, it's a struggle. When that happens, it's an opportunity for you to learn. Ask yourself 'OK, what was difficult about that, and what can I do to make it easier next time?'

There's no reason to stop after one day, either. If you left sugar out of your coffee for one day and found it easy, why would you go back to your old habit the next day?

ONE-WEEK EXPERIMENTS

One-day experiments start to let you see what you're capable of. One-week experiments build on that to give you a much better idea of how the activity you're doing makes you feel. The easiest way to conduct a one-week experiment is to simply replicate what you were doing for your one-day test – and do it seven times in a row.

When it comes to one-week experiments, there are several things you'll be looking for:

\# **How does it make you feel physically?** If you do a 20-minute walk every morning, how do you feel after each walk and at the end of each day? If you have a breakfast that is low in carbohydrate and high in good fats and protein, how do you feel at morning tea time? At lunch time? If you go to bed half an hour earlier than normal every day for a week, how does this affect your physical energy during the day? Note that if your experiment involves adding exercise to your day, be aware that this is not the time to be looking for gains in strength or aerobic fitness – that's going to take longer.

\# **How does it make you feel emotionally?** If you do a short deep-breathing or meditation exercise before you walk into the house after work, do you feel better able to cope with the demands of your kids? If you eliminate added sugars from your diet, how do you feel? Stressed, because you want them; or strong, because you know you're in control, not the sugar?

What thoughts go through your mind and threaten to derail you? Is there a voice saying 'I can't do this; there's no point; it's not going to make any difference, I might as well give up'? If there is, what can you say back to it, to make it shut up for a while?

With one-week experiments, you're usually trying to overcome a barrier or a habit. For example, if you know that you eat too much or frequently graze on delicious but unhealthy snacks, a one-week experiment can help you become more aware of your actions. You might start to ask yourself questions like 'Am I actually hungry, or is something else causing me to eat?' That 'something else' could be thirst, boredom, happiness, craving a sense of satisfaction, low energy, tiredness . . . There are lots of reasons why we reach for food, and most of them haven't got anything to do with hunger.

For most of these one-week experiments you can simply observe how you feel each day, and note the things you found challenging and how you felt each day. Be honest with yourself – if you found that eliminating all added sugars from your diet left you feeling grumpy and miserable, then maybe that target was too ambitious. You could be better to just cut back on the sugars for a while, rather than getting rid of them all at once.

ONE-MONTH EXPERIMENTS

Once you've got the hang of one-week experiments, it's time to tackle something with a bit more substance. Now you're looking at making a change and sustaining it for an entire month, to see what effect that has on your health.

For these longer experiments, you're looking for physical changes – looser clothes, more energy, better sleep, greater muscle strength, better mood. Again, you want to start with a clear baseline – so measure yourself before you begin your experiment. If you want, you can measure yourself every week to check your progress, or you can simply take measurements at the start and end of the experiment.

Measuring yourself too frequently isn't a good idea. Your body will vary naturally from day to day, so it's difficult to see a change over a short time. Think about your weight – if you're dehydrated because you spent all day at the beach and didn't have any drinks with you, then you'll weigh less than normal. But that's not weight loss – as soon as you rehydrate, you'll be back to where you started. (The 'lose 7 kilos in 7 days!' diets that litter the internet and magazines take advantage of this fluid loss – it's totally unsustainable, and definitely unhealthy!)

You can do pretty much anything for a one-month experiment, but there are a couple of things to watch out for.

If your experiment involves increasing your physical activity, build up gradually. If you've never run before, don't suddenly try to run 10 km every day – or even every second day. You'll end up demoralised, damaged, or both. Instead, set a goal of 30 minutes of aerobic activity every day – start with a walk, then build up to a walk-jog sequence, then increase the ratio of jogging in that sequence until you get to the point where you can jog for 30 minutes. Even then, alternate jogging days and walking days so that your body has time to recover from the session that involves more effort.

If your experiment involves changing your diet radically, get some professional advice – preferably from a dietitian or a registered nutritionist. Examples of radical diet changes would be deciding to remove all gluten-containing foods, suddenly adopting a vegan diet, trying a FODMAP diet – or any other approach that means you're removing entire food groups from your diet. Big dietary changes like this could end up doing more harm than good unless you know what you're doing. (For smaller changes, like swapping your morning toast and cereal for the BEAST breakfast, there's no need to consult an expert.)

#32 HABIT HELPERS

Setting new habits – or breaking old ones – is hard! If it was easy, the world would be full of happy, healthy people who regularly put money in their retirement account, brushed their teeth twice a day and made the bed every morning.

But despite it being hard, there are plenty of people around who have successfully changed what they do – and sustained that change. Some of them might have been forced to change, but for many others it will have been a choice. If you're making a choice to make a change, here are some tips that will make it a lot easier for you to stick to your new habits.

MAKE SURE YOU WANT TO CHANGE

If you don't have a strong 'why' – a strong reason for changing – then you don't have anything to fall back on when things get tough. Take a look at page 27 for ideas about finding your 'why' for change. Make sure that it's *you* who wants to change, too. If you're trying to make a change because someone else thinks you should, your chances of success are so much lower.

And make sure that the goal that you're setting is realistic – if your goal is to never eat sugar again but you know that sweet treats give you a lot of pleasure, then you're probably not ready to commit to that goal. If you feel the need for a big, final blow-out before you start your change, then maybe your goal isn't realistic. If you've decided to give up alcohol to improve your health but before you do that you're going to have a massive binge, then it's quite likely that you don't really want to give up alcohol at all, and cutting down would be a better goal.

PLAN YOUR START DATE

Don't just jump in and start immediately, tempting though that might be. You need to set up your environment so that it supports your goal. Decide that you're going to change, and what you're going to do, and then set your start date for a week or so in the future. This gives you time to get used to the idea, and it allows you to plan how you're going to tackle your goal. You'll have time to work out whether you *can* get up half an hour earlier to go for a walk, or if you *can* prepare extra dinner so that you've got leftovers to take in for lunch the next day.

CHANGE ONE HABIT AT A TIME

How many times have you made a bunch of New Year's resolutions and kept them for . . . oh, three days or so? Plenty? We all do it. On the first day of January, a lot of us decide we're going to revolutionise our lives – never eat junk food again, stop taking sugar in our tea or coffee, run every day, give up smoking, stop drinking, etc. And pretty much everyone who starts like this is on a fast-track to failure. It's impossible to change so much in so little time, because it takes willpower and attention. We only have a finite amount of willpower, and there's rarely enough to allow us to change everything.

Instead, pick just one thing to change. Just one. It might be to walk or run for 20 minutes every day. Maybe you want to try going to bed half an hour earlier so that you can get up 30 minutes earlier and do some exercise. Or perhaps you want to have a high-protein breakfast every day. Or to halve the amount of rice you eat. Whatever it is, make sure that there is just one thing you're trying to change.

When you're thinking about *which* change to make first, try choosing the one that will have the most impact, or the one that is most exciting to you, or the one that you think will be the easiest to achieve.

START SMALL

One of the biggest changes we've seen in the past couple of decades is the arrival of the internet. But that wasn't built overnight, you know. It started out as a few ugly pages – and just look at it now!

You can apply exactly the same idea to any change you want to make: start small, and gradually build up over time. So, if your change is to add exercise, go small to start with. If you can only do 5 minutes to start with, that's fine – just make sure you increase the time gradually so that you get to your goal. If you want to develop a healthier diet, try tackling just one meal a week to start with, then extend that to two meals the following week, etc.

Starting small makes it easy to achieve your goal to start with – this means that you get a good buzz from your accomplishments, and that way you're more likely to keep going.

BE ACCOUNTABLE

OK, so there's a voice inside your head saying that you're going to change. The problem is that only you can hear that voice, and what it has to say is transient and intangible. Worse still, there's another voice saying 'Nah, can't be bothered.' That voice is easier to listen to – because change is hard and it's human nature to choose the easy option and do what we've always done.

So, if you want to be successful at change and to stay on track, then you need an external way of recording your success. There are plenty of options here – pick one that works for you. You could keep a daily journal that you write in, you could have a 'healthy habits' buddy who you talk to every day, you could use an app to record your progress, you could put a big chalkboard up in the kitchen and tick off every day that you've followed your new habit. It doesn't matter which technique you use, as long as it feels right for you and you do it every day, ideally at the end of the day. If you don't have some sort of system like this to keep you accountable, you'll find that all of a sudden a week has gone by and you've lost the habit.

#33 PLAN TO SUCCEED

One of the tricks for adopting a healthier lifestyle is to find all the little opportunities in your day or week that help you change for the better. The key word here is 'little'. You don't need to suddenly magic up an extra six hours in your day to shop, cook, exercise, stretch and foam-roll your body into submission. You just need to tweak things that you already do. A few small steps, done regularly, will eventually bring about big changes.

Everyone's life is different, so we each have to work out our own tweaks. The following table shows some general ideas for one very common type of lifestyle – that of the working mum or dad. Although it might not exactly apply to your situation, it's a good example of the sorts of thing that happen – and how you can tweak them.

In this example, our mum (or dad) has been able to greatly increase their control over their diet just by taking a bit of time to plan what they are going to eat during the week. Spending a bit of time in the evening and on the weekend to make sure that they have easy options available when things are more rushed has really paid off. And they've also used some strategies to cope when they find themselves in situations where there's lots of tempting food – eating a bit less during the rest of the day, or taking a small portion and making it last, or choosing slightly healthier alternatives that still hit the spot. They've added in a little bit of exercise, some of it alone, and some of it with family. This is a great starting point and because it's not demanding unrealistic amounts of time, it's something that can be sustained.

ORIGINAL WEEK

	MORNING	DAY	EVENING
MONDAY	Crazy busy, organising kids, dashing to work; toast and jam eaten in the car.	Bought muffin for morning tea; sandwiches from café for lunch; picked up kids, did errands.	Something out of the freezer for dinner; crashed in front of TV with wine later on.
TUESDAY	Bit better than yesterday; cereal, yoghurt, juice for breakfast.	Banana from home for snack; bought sushi for lunch; took kids to friend's place after school.	Made spag bol for dinner, with salad and wine; went for a walk together; cheese and biscuits and more wine later on.
WEDNESDAY	Woke late; no time for breakfast.	Grazed on muesli bar and rice crackers all morning; starving – got burger and chips for lunch!	Cooked a proper meal. Ice creams all round afterwards; watched TV.
THURSDAY	Picked at leftovers from last night; took the rest into work for lunch.	Birthday shout at work – cake and biscuits.	Supermarket shop; pizza for dinner; couple of glasses of wine to recover.
FRIDAY	Kids fighting; barely managed to grab toast and honey for breakfast.	Our weekly day out for lunch – quiche and salad; shared a bit of chocolate cake.	Fish and chips for dinner, at the park by the beach.
SATURDAY	Kids to sports; grabbed breakfast from a takeaway van.	Just grazed through the day between housework and parenting duties!	Barbecue with friends; plenty of food – sausages, steak, garlic bread – and good wine, too.
SUNDAY	Much more relaxed start to the day; had some buttery croissants for breakfast.	Late lunch – well, just grazing again; cheese and crackers, fruit. Nice to just spend time at home as a family.	Cooked a nice dinner together; roast with quite a few of the trimmings!

TWEAKED WEEK

	MORNING	DAY	EVENING
MONDAY	Crazy busy, organising kids, dashing to work; took overnight oats to eat at work.	Tuna salad that was prepped on Sunday; 20-minute walk at lunchtime.	Made a curry with mince and packed it full of veg so it was nice and filling; glass of wine. Did some easy bodyweight exercises together while we watched TV.
TUESDAY	More time – made scrambled eggs on one slice of toast, plus avocado.	Leftover curry, plus some hummus and carrots for a snack.	Went for a walk together, then did a massive vege stir-fry with chicken.
WEDNESDAY	No time to cook – home-made muesli, yoghurt and blueberries.	A couple of no-pastry vege and cheese quiches made in muffin tins on Sunday; 20-minute walk at lunchtime.	Mid-week slump – resorted to sausages for dinner, but added veges (mostly frozen!). TV, but with some more bodyweight and flexibility exercises.
THURSDAY	The last of the overnight oats for the week.	Birthday shout at work – just took a small slice of cake and made it last! Quiche again.	Supermarket shop. Bought a cooked chicken and some fresh salads for an easy dinner.
FRIDAY	Kids fighting; still managed toast with sardines.	Our weekly day out for lunch – opted for a mix of two different salads and finished with a bliss ball to hit the sweet craving.	All on our bikes for a good ride, finishing up with fish and chips for dinner. Spent a couple of minutes making overnight oats for tomorrow's breakfast.
SATURDAY	Kids to sports; ate overnight oats while watching from the sideline.	Housework and parenting day! Omelette at lunchtime, zinged up with some leftover veg.	Barbecue with friends; indulged a bit but made sure to pile on the salads and kept it to just one piece of garlic bread!
SUNDAY	Nice cooked breakfast for everyone – went for the BEAST.	Got the kids to help with prepping breakfast and lunch options for the week.	Roast, no spuds but pumpkin and lots of other veges. Did extra veg so there would be some for the week.

TWELVE WEEKS, TWELVE TWEAKS

One way to transition to a more healthy lifestyle is to make a tweak a week. That might be one small change to your diet, or one to your level of exercise, or one to both aspects. It might be changing how or when you do something, so that you benefit from being more organised. It might be changing how much attention you pay to the voice inside your head, or how much you let other people influence your life.

If you want to take this approach, review the goals that you set earlier and identify some strategies that might help you achieve them. If you're not sure, use the experiment approach (see page 224) to help you get an idea of what might work. Then commit to the changes you're going to implement. Write them up on a big piece of paper or a chalkboard, or set them as reminders on your phone. If you've got family living with you, make sure they are in on the act too – otherwise they can scupper your chance of success before you even get going.

Here are some ideas for 12-week tweaks – choose them if they work for you, or design your own plan from scratch.

FOOD TWEAKS

WEEK	TWEAK	IS IT FOR YOU?
1	Reduce the amount of carbs on your plate.	
2	Add an extra non-starchy vegetable to dinner.	
3	Go without sandwiches for lunch all week.	
4	Stop putting sugar in your tea or coffee.	
5	Cook extra for dinner and have leftovers for lunch.	
6	Have three different-coloured veges at each dinner.	
7	Try a new vegetable each day.	
8	Have a portion of veges at breakfast.	
9	Try two new whole grains this week (e.g. barley, quinoa, amaranth, black rice, red rice, millet).	
10	Include a portion – or more – of veges with your lunch.	
11	Design three different quick but sustaining breakfasts that work for you.	
12	Go for a whole week without buying any ready-made food (includes bakery, sushi, frozen chips – but not frozen veg).	

EXERCISE TWEAKS

WEEK	TWEAK	IS IT FOR YOU?
1	Park as far away from work as possible every day.	
2	Take the stairs, not the elevator or escalator, every day.	
3	Do the '10-minute kickers' (page 104) every day.	
4	Get 150 minutes of aerobic exercise in the week.	
5	Walk for 10 minutes before work, at lunchtime and after work, every day.	
6	Do some type of physical exercise every time the adverts come on the TV.	
7	Try a new exercise activity – alone or with friends or family.	
8	Do squats while you brush your teeth.	
9	Get up 30 minutes earlier and exercise before starting the rest of your day.	
10	Spend 30 minutes each day energetically cleaning your house.	
11	Do mobility exercises while you're talking on the phone (use the speaker function so your hands are free).	
12	Get up and go for a walk at work every 30 minutes.	

OTHER TWEAKS

WEEK	TWEAK	IS IT FOR YOU?
1	Shop with a grocery list and stick to it.	
2	Pre-portion treats so you're less likely to overeat them.	
3	Plan your week's meals ahead, then stick to the plan.	
4	Dedicate some weekend time to meal prep and if you have family at home, get them involved.	
5	Buy suitable containers to keep prepared meals in the fridge or freezer.	
6	Try a new hobby if you think boredom leads you to overeat.	
7	Have a competition to see how many healthy meals or foods you can eat in a week.	
8	Limit TV time to an hour a night – use the saved time to do something that supports your healthy lifestyle.	
9	Go to bed 30 minutes earlier so you wake up more refreshed.	
10	Start a vege garden – grow your own food.	
11	Start a support group – family, friends, neighbours – to share and spread the healthy lifestyle message.	
12	Believe in yourself!	

FUNCTIONAL FITNESS FOR ALL — EXTRAS

If you've never really exercised before, then you could be forgiven for thinking there's a secret language that is spoken only in gyms, yoga studios and CrossFit boot camps. And yes, there are a few bits of lingo that you'll want to understand before you dive in to your new, health-focused lifestyle.

Engage your core: This is nothing to do with marriage proposals and everything to do with stability. Your core is basically the muscles around your torso, from your ribs down to your hips. These muscles stabilise your body and help you maintain good posture. If you spend a lot of time sitting, they can get a bit slack and forget to work. So, we need to make sure that they are paying attention when we do exercise – which means we need to engage them. To engage your core, lightly suck in your belly button so that it moves towards your spine. You will feel the muscles all around it tighten just slightly – now they are switched on and engaged and ready to keep you stable while you move. Be sure to keep the movement light – you want to feel the muscles contract a bit, but there shouldn't be any sense of stress with the contraction.

Switch on your glutes/back muscles/etc: This is very similar to engaging your core. You want to lightly contract the muscles so that they help to stabilise you, or so that they are ready for a bigger challenge, for example, if you're about to lift a heavy weight.

Move with control: Think of a ballet dancer – when they dance, their movement is controlled and deliberate.

When you're exercising, try to move with similar control. If you're lowering a weight (even if that weight is your body), do it in a deliberate, controlled manner. That will work your muscles properly and reduce the chance of you getting an injury.

\# **Neutral spine:** Your spine has a natural curve to it – a slight S shape, if viewed from the side. When your spine is resting like this, it's in neutral, which is its strongest, healthiest position. Prolonged sitting can leave some people with a spine that doesn't sit in neutral naturally. If you're not sure what neutral feels like, try this: lie on the floor on your back, with your knees bent. There should be a natural hollow under your lower spine and you should be able to slip your hand in there. To check, try tilting your pelvis back and forward. When you tilt your pelvis back, your spine will go flat on the floor. When you tilt forward, you will create an even bigger gap under your spine. The neutral spot that you are looking for is where your pelvis is neither tilted forward nor back, but sits level.

\# **A note on your neck:** Our over-abundance of screen time these days means a lot of people are developing a habit of sticking their neck forward, which puts a huge strain on neck muscles and can lead to tension headaches and other problems. If you know you do this, try to be conscious of keeping your chin tucked in when you are exercising. At the same time, be aware of your neck muscles and make sure that you're not tightening them up when you're doing these exercises – you don't need to use your neck muscles to lift a weight!

\# **Breathing:** This is important – and people often forget to do it when they are concentrating on an exercise. As a general rule, breathe out on the effort part of an exercise, and breathe in on the easy part. For example, breathe out on the push part of a push-up, and breathe in as you lower yourself down to the floor. Don't worry if you get it wrong or you're not sure which part of an exercise is the effort part – just keep breathing!

HOW TO DO IT

- # Pick one exercise from each of the five categories – push, pull, hip-hinge, squat and pillar.
- # Do 10–12 reps (repetitions) of each, with a minute or so of recovery time between each exercise.
- # Repeat this twice, so that you've done a total of three sets.

Do this three or four times a week for the best results.

A WORD OF CAUTION

If you haven't done anything like this before, start with the easiest option and do just a few reps. The worst thing you can do is believe that you're ready for the advanced exercises right from the get-go – and most of us think this way. If you begin at a higher level than your body can tolerate, you'll quickly lose form and will risk injuring yourself. Focus on the *journey* at the start – you will soon find that you can move on to more demanding versions of the exercises, and that will give you a nice sense of achievement.

Correct form is paramount. Regardless of your level, you should stop your repetitions when you have fatigued or reached technical failure. That is, you can no longer hold perfect form and you are trying to cheat some more reps!

PUSH EXERCISES

Push exercises can be used to build both strength and stability in your upper and lower body. Even without any extra gear, you can build up your leg and hip strength with lunges, and your arm, shoulder and chest strength with push-ups. At the same time, you will be adding to your core stability – all without a single sit-up! If you find that lunges cause you a bit of knee pain, reduce the distance of your forward step and then gradually increase it as you get stronger. If forward lunges cause issues, try reverse lunges instead, as these are often easier for people with dodgy knees.

BODYWEIGHT BASIC — NO GEAR NEEDED

LUNGES - WITH VARIATIONS

STATIC LUNGE

Stand upright, shoulders back, core engaged and chin up. Pick a point a few metres in front of you to focus on – this will stop you looking down during the lunge.

Step one leg forward, lowering your hips until both knees are bent to a 90-degree angle. Make sure that your front knee is directly above your ankle and in line with your third or fourth toe. Check that your other knee doesn't touch the floor.

To rise up, push down through your heel and use the strength in your glutes and quads. Don't take a step back; sink down into the lunge again and repeat until you have completed your exercise set.

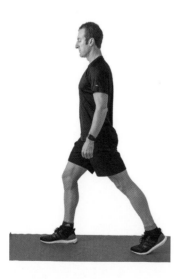 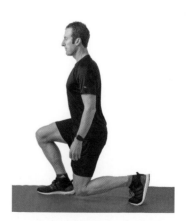

FORWARD LUNGE

Follow the instructions for the static lunge, but once you have lowered your body and have both knees at a 90-degree angle,

return to the starting position by pushing down evenly through your front foot and taking a controlled step back so that you are standing upright.

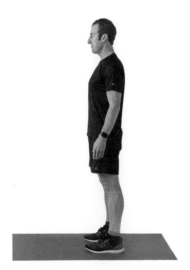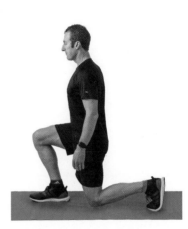

REVERSE LUNGE

Follow the instructions for the forward lunge, but instead of taking a step forward, take a step backwards.

To return to the starting position, push down through the rear foot and take a controlled step forward so that you are standing upright.

WALKING LUNGE

Follow the instructions for the forward lunge, but instead of taking a step back to return to the starting position, lunge forward with the other leg, so that you are travelling forward in a series of lunges on alternate legs.

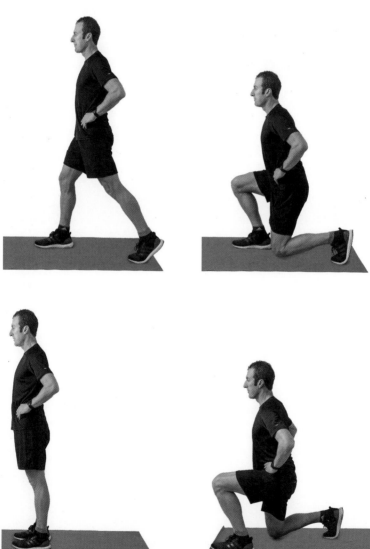

SIDE LUNGE

Stand upright, legs slightly wider than shoulder-distance apart, and toes pointed forward.
Shift your bodyweight onto one leg, and bend that knee until it reaches a 90-degree angle and the other leg is straight. Control the movement with your quads and your glutes.
Push down through the bent leg to raise your body and return to the starting position, then repeat on the other side.

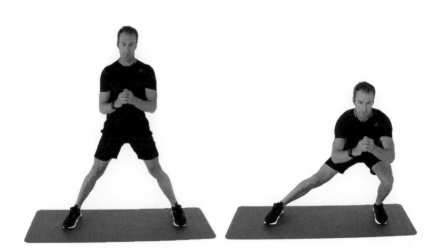

BULGARIAN SPLIT SQUAT

Stand on your right leg, with your left foot resting on a bench or box behind you.
Bend your right knee, lowering your body until your left knee is hovering just above the ground.
Straighten your right leg (try not to push off the rear leg) to complete one rep.
Do all the reps on one side before switching legs.

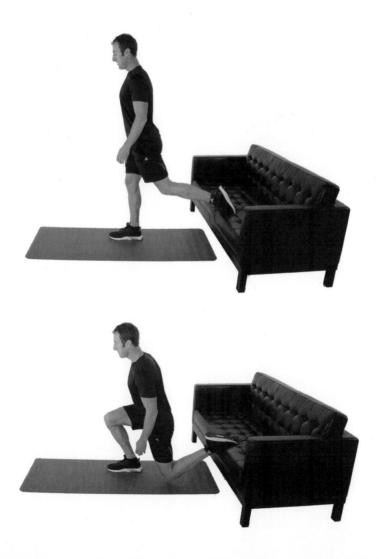

PUSH-UPS - WITH VARIATIONS

CLASSIC PUSH-UP

Lie face down on the ground, and put your hands flat on the ground at shoulder height and slightly wider than shoulder-width apart. Find a hand position that feels comfortable for you – your middle finger can point forward away from you, or your hands can rotate inwards slightly if that feels better for your wrists. (If you're on a semi-soft surface like carpet or grass, you can also do push-ups on your knuckles.)

Set your feet at a width that feels right for you: doing push-ups with your feet together is more challenging than doing them with your feet wide apart.

Look ahead, not down. Lightly engage all of the muscles in your core and glutes, then push up so that your arms are straight. You want to be able to keep the whole of your body in a straight line all the way through this movement. If your butt is sticking up in the air or you're sagging down through the middle, you're not using enough core strength.

To start the actual push-up, lower yourself down with control, keeping your elbows tucked in to your body. If they start to fly out, you're getting too tired. Ideally you will be able to lower yourself so that your arms are bent to 90 degrees. If you can go lower – e.g. so that your chest touches the floor – that's great.

Pause at the bottom of the movement, then push back up to complete one repetition.

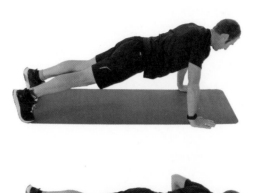

KNEELING PUSH-UP

This is an easier variation, and a good place to start if you haven't done push-ups before. The action is the same as the classic push-up, except that you are resting on your knees rather than your toes. This reduces the amount of bodyweight that you need to move, and allows you to develop good form before you move to full-body push-ups.

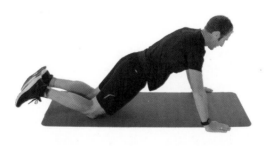

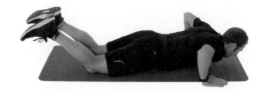

ELEVATED PUSH-UP VARIATIONS

These are variations that are slightly easier than the classic push-up, and help you maintain good form while you build strength. Instead of having your hands on the floor, use a couch or a hard suitcase (make sure it can't scoot away from you!). Since you're not taking your body all the way down to the ground, you don't have to work quite so hard.

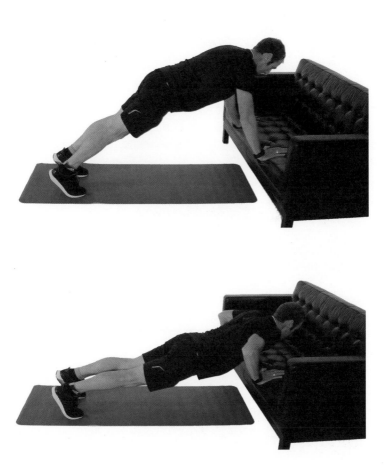

HAND-RELEASE PUSH-UP

This slows the overall motion of the push-up, and stops any cheating!

Start with a classic push-up, but lower your body to the floor, let your chest touch the ground, and lift your hands up so they aren't touching the ground. You can lift your hands backwards by pinching your shoulder blades together; or, if that's too tiring, just rock them forwards a bit. Whichever way you choose, make sure that you completely break contact with the ground.

Put your hands back on the ground and perform the next push-up.

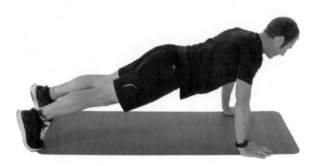

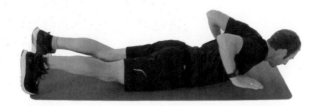

PIKE PUSH-UP

This is a harder push-up than the classic version. Start in a downward dog position, so that your body is like an inverted V, with your butt in the air and your feet and hands on the ground. Your arms will be positioned forward of your shoulders.

Lower your upper body by bending your arms at the elbow, then press back up to complete one rep.

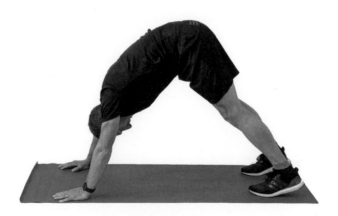

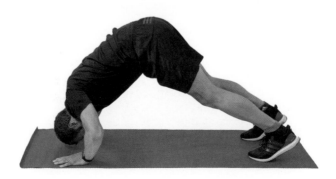

WALL PUSH-UP

This is only for push-up experts! Do not attempt this unless you are very proficient at push-ups.

Kneel in front of a wall, facing away from it, with your arms straight down in front of you at shoulder width and your hands on the ground (standard four-point kneeling).

Slide your feet up the wall so that you are in a handstand position, then complete push-ups, allowing your feet to travel up and down the wall with the movement.

SINGLE-LEG PUSH-UP

This is another advanced push-up and should only be attempted once you are very good at classic push-ups.

Set yourself up exactly as you would for a classic push-up, then engage your glutes and hamstrings to raise one leg. Make sure that you're using your glutes, and not putting stress on your back muscles.

Perform push-ups with the leg raised throughout, then swap and do the other side.

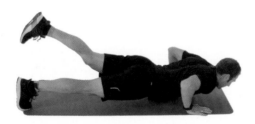

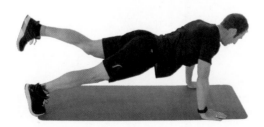

BODYWEIGHT PLUS – ADD SOME SIMPLE GEAR

LUNGES

All of the lunges described in the previous section can be made more challenging by adding some weight or by incorporating a resistance band.

- # If adding weight, start with something relatively light (a tin of food or a full water bottle in each hand), and build up from there.
- # To use a resistance band with these exercises, wrap the band around your back and secure the ends so that as you rise from the lunge you have to work against the tension in the band.

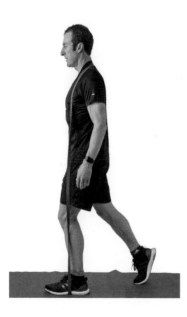
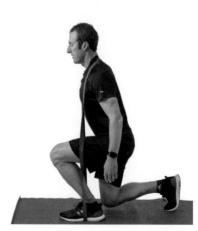

PUSH-UPS

To increase the difficulty of the push-ups, either move to a more difficult variation or add some resistance or weight. You could put a weight on your back (make sure it's something that's not going to slip off), or you could wrap a resistance band over your upper back and pin it to the ground with your hands, so that when you push up you are working against the tension in the band.

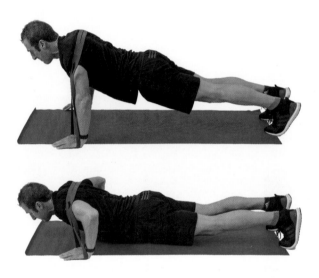

FULL NOISE – WELL-EQUIPPED HOME GYM OR COMMERCIAL GYM

LUNGES AND BULGARIAN SPLIT SQUAT

The Bulgarian split squat and all of the lunges described in the previous section can be made more challenging by adding weight in the form of dumbbells or barbells. Start out with lighter weights and increase the weight slowly.

It's important to maintain good form when you include weights with these exercises. If using a barbell, position it behind your back so that it rests across your shoulders – don't let the weight rest on your neck. It's worth getting your form checked by an expert – the last thing you want to do is to injure yourself.

BENCH PRESS

Lie face up on a bench, holding a heavy barbell at your sternum, your hands shoulder-width apart and your elbows bent into your sides.

Extend your arms, pushing the bar directly above your chest. Pause, then lower the barbell to complete a single rep.

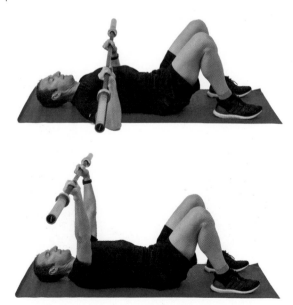

DUMBBELL SHOULDER PRESS

ARNIE PRESS

This is the way that Arnold Schwarzenegger used to do shoulder presses. Don't try this variation if you have rotator cuff problems.

Start (sitting or standing as for the standard press) by holding the dumbbells out in front of you, arms bent to 90 degrees at shoulder height, and hands rotated inwards so you are looking at your wrists.

As you start to push up, open your shoulders and rotate your wrists and straighten your arms, so that at the top of the movement, the dumbbells are touching overhead in the same position as the standard dumbbell press.

Reverse the movement, with control, to return to the starting position.

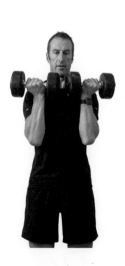
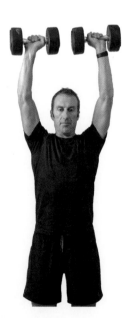

SHOULDER PRESS

This is similar to the Arnie press, but start with hands palms out just outside shoulder width, and press up to the same finish position.

   #   Sit on a bench with back support. (You can also do this exercise standing, or sitting on a bench without a back, although if you have lower back problems then it's best to use back support.) Hold a dumbbell in each hand, resting them upright on your thighs.

   #   To get to the starting position, raise your arms so that they are bent at 90 degrees, with your elbows at shoulder height, your palms facing forward and the dumbbells horizontal. (If the dumbbells are heavy, use your thighs to bounce them up.)

   #   As you breathe out, press up with your arms, raising the dumbbells so that they nearly touch over your head.

   #   Pause briefly to breathe in, then breathe out as you lower your arms, with control, to the starting position to complete one repetition.

PULL EXERCISES

BODYWEIGHT BASIC – NO GEAR NEEDED

TYIW SERIES

This is a great series of movements that you can use to improve your shoulder health. It targets the rotator cuff, scapular and thoracic muscle groups. You can do these either lying face down on the floor, or standing with your knees bent slightly and your body bent forward at the hips so that your torso is parallel to the floor.

- # **T** Start with your arms hanging straight down, raise your arms out to the side of your body to form a T shape. Your thumbs should be pointing up.
- # **Y** From the same starting position, thumbs facing forward, raise your arms in front of your body to form a Y shape. Your thumbs should be pointing up.
- # **I** From the same starting position, raise your arms straight out in front of your body.
- # **W** From the same starting position, bend your elbows and lift your arms so that the upper part of each arm is tucked in next to your ribcage.
  Squeeze your shoulder blades together, and at the same time rotate your lower arms at the elbow, so that your hands go out and your arms form a W shape. Your elbows should stay tucked in to your body.

To start with, do 8 reps of each of the four exercises in a continuous fashion (32 reps in total). To progress, simply complete more sets e.g. 2-3 times through with 2 minute rests (3x32 reps).

T

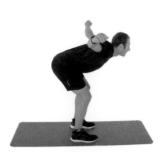
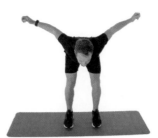

Y

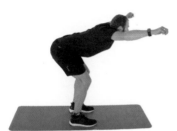
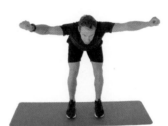

I

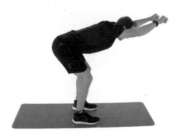
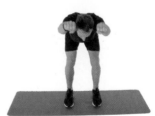

W

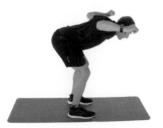
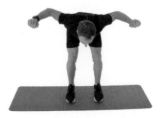

PULL-UP

It's challenging to do a pull-up without some sort of gear – but you don't have to go out and buy anything. Check out your local park – is there a kid's climbing frame or other equiptment there? Some parks also have a range of exercise equipment that's suitable. If yes, try some pull-ups. (You could also try these on a solid, stable bench or table at home.)

Choose a bar that's reasonably high but that you can reach without difficulty. With your palms facing towards you, hang from the bar with your arms straight and your knees bent so that your feet don't touch the ground.

Bend your elbows and pull your chest towards the bar. Then, slowly lower yourself down to complete one rep.

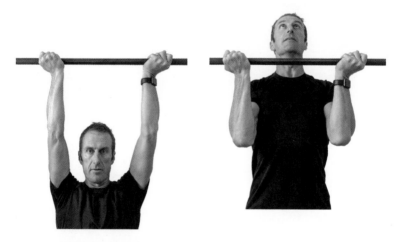

HORIZONTAL PULL-UP

This exercise needs a strong, stationary fitting for you to hold on to, like a door or ladder.

Open the door and stand facing it, with your feet either side. Take hold of both door handles and lean back, keeping your elbows tucked in close to your body.

Make sure that your core is engaged, so that your body is in a straight line – don't let yourself sag at the waist or hips, or round through the shoulders. As you breathe out,

bring your shoulder blades together while pulling your body towards the door.

Breathe in as you lower yourself, with control, back to the starting position.

If you have a staircase with strong, open bannisters (or a similar structure), you can wrap a towel around the bannisters and hold on to both ends with your hands, then lean back into the starting position, and repeat the movement described above.

The greater the angle of your body (i.e. the closer you are to horizontal, rather than vertical), the more challenging the movement.

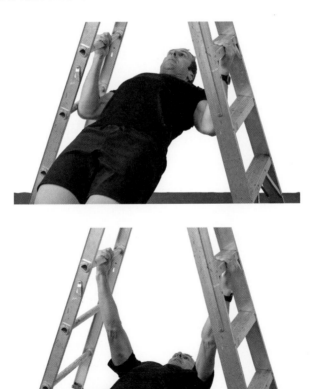

BODYWEIGHT PLUS – ADD SOME SIMPLE GEAR

All of the pull exercises described above can be made more challenging by adding some weight. Start with light weights – this is especially important for the TYIW series. Going for more weight than your body can handle will greatly increase the chances of you getting an injury, so don't do it! Remember, form is king.

FULL NOISE – WELL-EQUIPPED HOME GYM OR COMMERCIAL GYM

PULL-UP
  # With your palms facing away from you, hang from a bar with your arms straight and your knees bent so that your feet don't touch the floor.
  # Bend your elbows, pulling your chest towards the bar. Slowly lower yourself, with control, to complete one rep.

DUMBBELL ROW
  # Put a dumbbell on the floor to the left of a bench, then stand at one end of that bench, on the same side as the dumbbell. Place your right knee on the bench, bend from the hips so that your upper body is parallel to the floor, and place your right hand on the other end of the bench.
  # Keeping your lower back straight, use your left hand to grasp the dumbbell, with your palm facing your body. As you breathe out, use your back muscles to pull your left arm up to the side of your chest. Your torso should remain stationary, and your forearms shouldn't do any work other than holding on to the dumbbell – the movement comes from the contraction of your back muscles: squeeze these as you reach the top of the movement.

- # As you breathe out, lower the weight with control, to complete one rep. Repeat the exercise on the other side.
- # As a variation, dumbbell rows can be done using a high or low pulley, rather than the dumbbell.

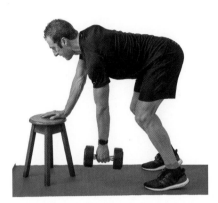 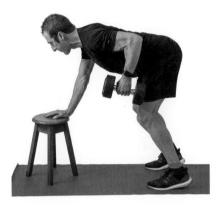

SUSPENSION TRAINER ROW

BEGINNER LEVEL

- # Stand in front of a suspension trainer, holding the handles in front of you. Raise your arms so that they are straight above your head, and cross one foot over the other. Lean back slightly and bend your elbows out to the side at the same time.
- # To do the row, pull your body up towards your hands. Pause, then lower your body, with control, to the starting point.

INTERMEDIATE LEVEL

- # Stand in front of a suspension trainer, holding the handles in front of you. With both feet on the floor, lean back 60 degrees and bend your knees while pulling your elbows out to the side.
- # Keeping your body as straight as possible, pull yourself back to the starting position.

ADVANCED LEVEL

  # Sit on the floor in front of a suspension trainer, holding the handles in front of you. Your legs should be straight so that your body is shaped like the letter L, with your arms above your head.

  # Bending your elbows, pull your body up towards your hands, keeping your upper body as vertical as possible. Pause, then lower your body to the starting position. Note that most suspension straps can support 130–150 kg of bodyweight; set them to the highest level for this exercise and if you are at the upper end of this bodyweight range, use anchors to ensure your safety. This is particularly important for the advanced level, as this will put the most weight/force on the suspension trainer fittings.

LAT PULLDOWN

  # Stand facing a lat pulldown machine, and grab hold of the bar over your head, with your arms just outside shoulder width and your wrists facing either away or towards you.

  # Lightly engage your back muscles, and stabilise your shoulders by pulling your shoulder blades together and down towards your back pockets.

  # Squeeze your lats to bring the bar down to your chin. Don't pull the bar behind your neck, as this reduces the range of motion of your lats. Don't pull the bar down below your chest, as this can make your shoulders come forward and cause problems, especially if you already have cranky shoulders. Gripping too wide will also cause shoulder irritation.

  # Keep the weights light to begin with – if you need to use momentum to pull the bar down, then you have too much weight loaded and will not be targeting your lats.

SEATED ROW

  # Sit on a seated row machine with your feet on the front platform or crossbar, and your knees slightly bent. Lean

forward and grasp the handles. Keeping your arms extended, pull back until your torso is at a 90-degree angle to your legs. This is your starting position: your back should be slightly arched, your chest should be sticking out, and you should feel a nice stretch on your lats.

\# Keeping your torso stationary, breathe out as you pull the handles back towards your body until you are touching your abs, keeping your arms close to your sides throughout the movement.

\# Hold briefly, then breathe in as you slowly return to the starting position. Avoid swinging your torso back and forth during this exercise, as doing this can cause a lower back injury.

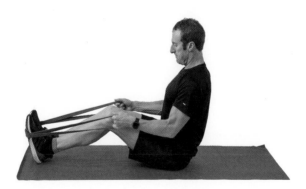

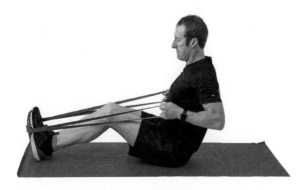

HIP-HINGE EXERCISES

Your hips are a really important pair of joints. You need to have strong, stable yet flexible hips for all sorts of activities – even walking. If you're only 30 you might not think that your hips are important – but just look at an older person who walks stiffly or who is bent over, and you'll get an idea of how wrong you are! We spend so much time sitting these days that our hip strength, flexibility and range of motion all suffer. Spend some time reversing this effect, and you won't regret it.

BODYWEIGHT BASIC – NO GEAR NEEDED

GOOD MORNING
This is essentially a controlled bow.
   # Stand with your feet hip-width apart, and your knees slightly bent. Hold your arms by your side. Lightly contract your back muscles, pulling your shoulder blades together and down, as though they were heading for your back pockets.
   # Keeping your back in neutral, bend forward at the hips. Push your hips back behind you, maintaining control throughout the movement. You should be able to get your upper body close to parallel with the floor.
   # To come back up, use the strength in your hamstring and glute muscles to raise your body – don't use your back muscles! Your arms should stay by your side throughout the movement.

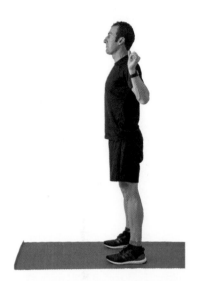
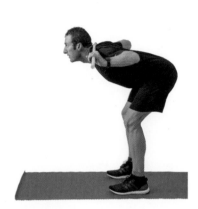

SINGLE-LEG ROMANIAN DEADLIFT

\# Stand on your right leg and hold your left arm so that it is in front of your left thigh. Have your left leg slightly bent and keep it in line with your body throughout the movement – don't let it drift off to the left or right.

\# Move your hips back as if you were being pulled by a rope around your waist; allow your right knee to bend slightly. Keeping your back in neutral, continue to bend forward at the hip while allowing your left leg to rise up behind you as a counterbalance. Ideally, your upper body will end up close to parallel with the floor and your left hand will be about mid-shin height (measured against your right leg).

\# To come back up, push down through your right heel and use the strength in your hamstrings and glutes to raise your body; push your hips forward to return to the starting position. Complete your reps for one side, then change legs and do the other side.

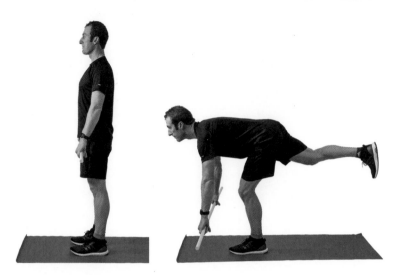

HIP THRUST

If you have a low couch, bench or chair, sit on the ground in front of it, with your back to it. If you don't have anything suitable, just lie flat on the ground. Bend your knees, with your feet flat on the floor.

If you have a couch, lean back so that your shoulder blades rest on it. From either position, push down through your feet to lift your hips up. All of your weight should be on your shoulder blades and your feet. Push your hips up as high as you can, using the strength in your glutes and hamstrings.

Hold briefly, then lower your hips in a controlled manner and return to the starting position.

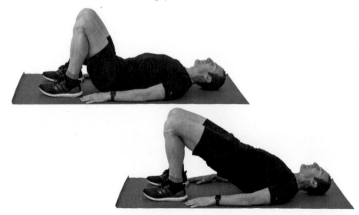

FROG SQUAT

\# Stand with your legs a bit wider than shoulder-width apart. Push your bottom back and bend your knees, grab hold of your toes and press your elbows to the inside of each knee. This is your starting position.

\# Push down through your feet into the floor and straighten your legs as far as you can. Your bottom will swing up and your upper body will tilt down towards the floor.

\# Return to the starting position and repeat for the desired number of repetitions.

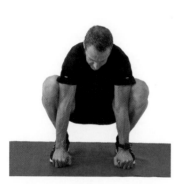
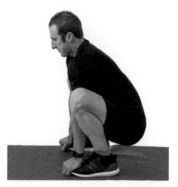
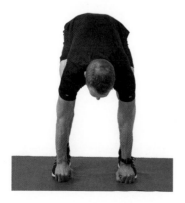
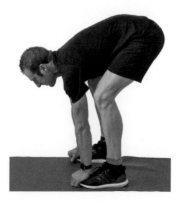

BODYWEIGHT PLUS – ADD SOME SIMPLE GEAR

GOOD MORNING

Make this harder by holding a weight (kettlebell, dumbbell, heavy brick, 2-litre bottle of water). Or, wrap a resistance band around your back and stand on the ends so that as you move back to the starting position, you have to work against the tension of the band.

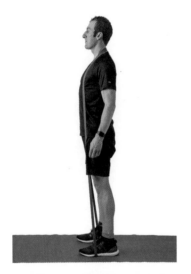
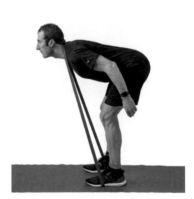

SINGLE-LEG ROMANIAN DEADLIFT

Make this harder by holding a small weight (light dumbbell, tin of food, bottle of water) or by using a resistance band.

DID YOU KNOW?

The average age of a muscle cell is 15 years – but your old cells are constantly being replaced with new ones.

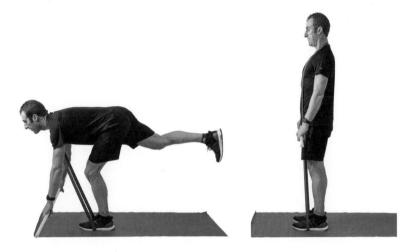

HIP THRUST

Make this harder by balancing a weight (securely) over your hips. Or, place a resistance band across your hips and hold it down on the floor with your feet or hands, so that as you raise your hips you have to work against the tension of the band.

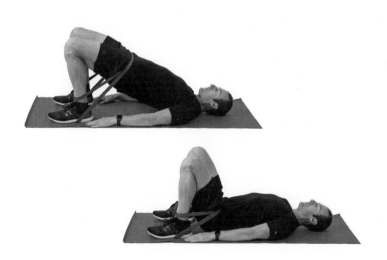

FULL NOISE — WELL-EQUIPPED HOME GYM OR COMMERCIAL GYM

DEADLIFT WITH BARBELL

Set a heavy barbell on the floor in front of you. Push your hips back and hinge at the hip, bending your knees slightly. Grip the bar at a bit wider than shoulder width, with your palms facing your body.

While maintaining a strong, neutral back, push your feet down into the floor to move into a standing position. To avoid stress on your lower back, keep your chest out and your spine in neutral, and keep the bar as close to your body as possible (even so that it slides up and down your legs).

Slowly lower the bar, with control, to complete one rep.

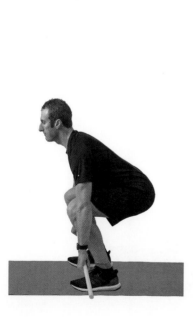
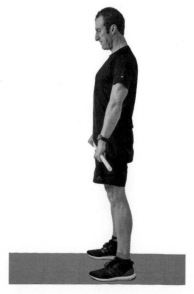

KETTLEBELL SWING

\# Stand with your feet hip-width apart and hold a kettlebell in front of you with your arms fully extended and your elbows soft – neither locked nor bent. Make sure that your back is in neutral and your core is engaged.

\# Lightly contract your back muscles so that your shoulder blades move together and down, as though they were heading for your back pockets. This will stop you rounding your shoulders and upper back.

\# Bend your knees slightly, then push your body forward from the hips to initiate the kettlebell swing. Swing the kettlebell to chest height, being sure not to lift your shoulders up – don't let them creep towards your ears.

\# Let momentum swing the kettlebell back down and between your legs as you hinge at the hips to continue the movement into the second swing. Stay in control by keeping your core engaged.

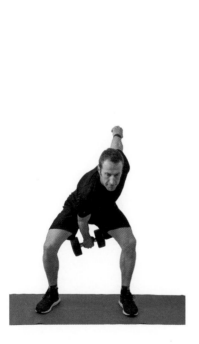
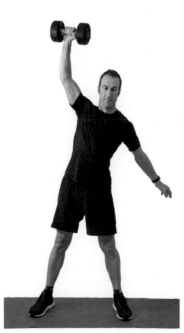

ROMANIAN DEADLIFT WITH BARBELL

Stand with both feet on the ground, shoulder-width apart, holding a barbell in both hands in front of your body, wrists facing you.

Move your hips back as if you were being pulled by a rope around your waist, allowing your knees to bend slightly. Keep your back in neutral, making sure not to round through your upper back, and bend forwards at the hips until the barbell is at about mid-shin height.

To return to the start position, push down through your heels and use the strength in your hamstrings and glutes to raise your body and push your hips forward.

Maintain control throughout the entire movement.

BARBELL HIP THRUST

This is the same as a regular hip thrust, except that you add some extra resistance by placing a weighted barbell across your hips. You might want to use some padding! Hold on to the barbell with your hands to stop it from rolling back and injuring you. Practise the movement without weights until you can do it easily, and as you progress, only add a small amount of weight each time.

DID YOU KNOW?

All of the blood in your body travels through your heart in the space of 1 minute.

SQUAT EXERCISES

If there is one exercise that really delivers bang for buck, it's the squat. Done properly, a squat will test your ability to move through your ankles, knees, hips, back and shoulders. It works a wide range of muscles, including your hamstrings, quads, glutes, core, back and more.

It's important to realise that because we are all built slightly differently, what looks like a perfect squat for one person might not be the same for another person. If you have a long femur (thigh bone), your squat will look different to one done by a person with a relatively short femur. On top of that, most of us have got some sort of movement restriction that makes achieving the perfect squat difficult. If you keep working on your mobility, though, your squat will eventually improve.

BODYWEIGHT BASIC — NO GEAR NEEDED

Stand with your feet shoulder-width apart, with your weight evenly distributed. Make sure that you're not gripping the floor with your toes – you should be able to wiggle these throughout the entire movement. Check that your back is straight, your spine is in neutral and your core is engaged. Extend your arms in front of you to act as a counterbalance.

Breathe in, then move out of your upright stance by pushing your hips back. As your hips travel further back, start to bend at the knees. Beginners often bend at the knees first – make sure that your hips lead the movement! Keep your chest and shoulders up, and keep looking straight ahead. Focus on keeping your knees in line with your feet. If they start to drift inwards, push them out so they track with your feet, but don't let them go wider than your feet – your knees and toes should be in line with each other.

281

\# To complete a full squat, you need to squat down until your hip joint is lower than your knees – for most people, this will be when their thighs are parallel to the ground. If you're really good at squatting, you may be able to go deeper.

\# To return to the start position, push down through your heels and use the strength in your glutes to raise your body. Breathe out as you do this. Make sure that the balls of your feet stay on the ground and that your knees stay in line with your toes all the way up to standing.

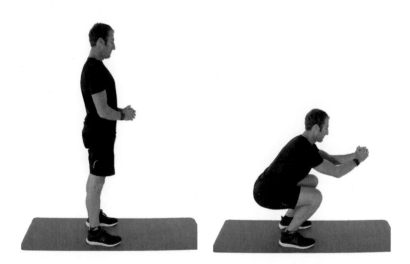

BODYWEIGHT PLUS – ADD SOME SIMPLE GEAR

Once you have mastered the basic squat, you can begin to challenge yourself by adding some weight or using a resistance band. The weight can be a few kilos – a medicine ball is great, if you have one, but you could also use a decent-sized brick or old patio tile. It just needs to be something you can hold comfortably in both hands. If you're going to use a resistance band, stand on it with both feet and hold one end in each hand or hook over your shoulders. Adjust the length so that when you stand up, you will be working against the tension in the band.

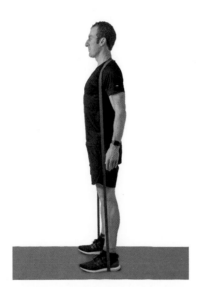
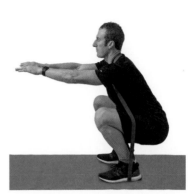

FULL NOISE – WELL-EQUIPPED HOME GYM OR COMMERCIAL GYM

To stretch yourself in a gym, place a barbell (with light weights to start off with) across your back and hold on to it with both hands. Make sure that the barbell is well away from your neck – the lower down across your shoulders you can position it, the better. Then do your squats, maintaining good technique and control throughout.

PILLAR EXERCISES

Pillar exercises like the plank strengthen the core (rib cage to hips), as well as the shoulders and upper back.

BODYWEIGHT BASIC – NO GEAR NEEDED

PLANK AND VARIATIONS

Plank-style exercises come in a number of variations with different levels of challenge, and can be performed anywhere, any time. All variations can be made a bit easier or a bit more difficult, depending on how strong your core is.

HIGH PLANK

Lie face down on the floor, with your palms on the floor next to your shoulders and your feet flexed so that you are up on your toes.

Breathe in, then as you breathe out press up into a push-up while drawing your navel towards your spine and tightening your glutes; don't let your lower back sag. Your body should form a straight line from your heels to the top of your head. Keep your head in a neutral position by looking at the floor.

Hold for at least 10 seconds, breathing normally, then lower yourself back to the floor in a controlled manner.

DID YOU KNOW?

Prolonged lack of sleep can cause your heartbeat to become irregular.

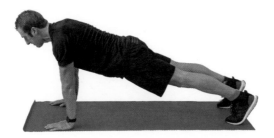

LOW PLANK

This is the same as the high plank except that your elbows are on the floor directly beneath your shoulders, with your hands clasped in front of your face so that your forearms make an inverted V.

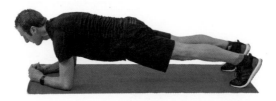

SIDE PLANK

Start in the low plank position, then rotate your body to the right and balance on your right arm, with your left foot stacked on top of your right foot. Your left arm can either rest on your hip or be extended towards the ceiling.

Hold the plank for at least 10 seconds, then return to full plank and lower yourself back to the floor in a controlled manner.

Repeat on the other side.

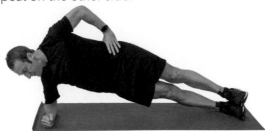

MAKE PLANKS EASIER

If you haven't done much core work in the past, then planks might be a bit of a challenge to start with. Reduce the intensity by doing planks from your knees rather than your toes (similar to doing push-ups off your knees). This will reduce the amount of weight that your body has to hold up, while helping you build the muscle strength that you need.

MAKE PLANKS MORE DIFFICULT

Once you're a plank expert, you can start to challenge yourself by lifting one leg off the ground during the plank, keeping it raised for half of your 'hold time', then switching and raising the other leg for the second half of your plank.

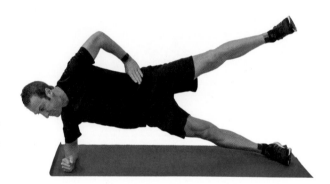

CRUNCH

Lie on your back with your knees slightly bent and your feet planted firmly on the floor, about hip-width distance apart. Don't let your knees sag inwards.

Fold your arms over your chest and tighten your abs, using the strength of these muscles to lift your head and shoulders off the floor. Hold for three deep breaths, then return to the starting position.

Keep your movements smooth and controlled, and stop if you lose form. Don't put your hands behind your head, as this puts your neck at risk of injury and stops you from effectively isolating your abs.

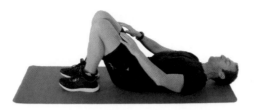

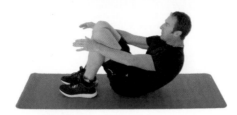

REVERSE CRUNCH

Lie on your back with your legs together, your knees slightly bent, your feet planted firmly on the floor, about hip-width distance apart, and your hands underneath your head.

Press your lower back into the floor and pull in your belly button to lift your feet off the floor – keep your knees together, bent to a 90-degree angle. Using your core, pull your knees into your chest so that your tailbone raises off the ground. At the same time, perform a traditional crunch by using your abs – not your hands! – to lift your head and shoulders so that your shoulder blades are off the floor.

Pause, then slowly lower your shoulders, hips and legs, stopping when your feet are just above the floor.

Repeat the movement without using momentum to power the next rep.

DID YOU KNOW?

If you exercise in the evening and then eat a high-protein meal, you will increase the amount of muscle your body builds while you are asleep.

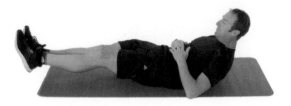

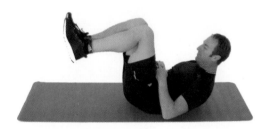

\# **Make it easier** – lower your feet all the way to the floor at the end of each rep, or simply reduce the height that you raise your shoulders and hips during the crunch.

\# **Make it harder** – instead of having your knees bent, keep your legs straight out in front of you, hovering just above the floor.

\# **Make it even harder** – have your legs straight out in front of you, then raise them overhead before using your abs to lift your hips off the floor. Finish the move by lowering your legs so that they are straight in front of you again, hovering just off the floor. Keep your shoulders lifted off the floor throughout the entire movement.

BODYWEIGHT PLUS – ADD SOME SIMPLE GEAR

The farmer's walk will test the integrity of your core while you're in a vertical stance. Stand up straight, holding a heavy weight in each hand with your palms facing towards your body. Walk 20 metres, maintaining your posture the whole time. Turn and walk back to the start point to complete one rep.

FULL NOISE – WELL-EQUIPPED HOME GYM OR COMMERCIAL GYM

The farmer's walk (see page 288) is especially suited to a gym where you can use heavy dumbbells for your weights.

DID YOU KNOW?

Your muscles burn energy even when you're just sitting on the couch watching TV. The more muscle you have, the more energy you'll burn.

BONUS EXERCISES

ROLLING

When we were babies we were able to roll over with minimal use of our legs or arms. We had a relatively heavy head, and used our central muscles to roll over. As adults, we don't tend to do this, but it's a great movement for testing your spinal musculature.

   \# Lie flat on your back with your arms stretched out over your head and your feet together. Tense your body a bit, and lift your hands and feet off the floor slightly.

   \# Turn your head and eyes in the direction that you want to roll, then reach your opposite arm across your body to initiate the movement, while turning your head into your shoulder at the same time. Roll onto your stomach, then reverse the movement and roll on to your back. Keep your body long and strong throughout the whole movement.

   \# To mix it up, try leading with your legs rather than your arms.

Note: Rolling should be nearly effortless, so if you find your upper back or neck muscles getting tight during the movement, then pause, breathe and relax. This is not a strength-training exercise. It's a restorative movement pattern that you should practise until you can do it easily. After that, you can move on to the next functional movement pattern, which is crawling.

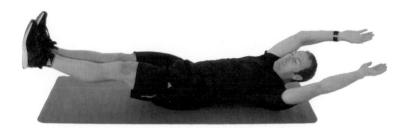

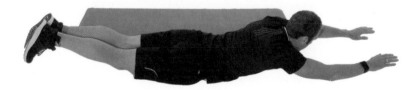

BABY CRAWL

- # Kneel on all fours, with your wrists under your shoulders and your knees under your hips.
- # Keeping your back in neutral, pull your belly button towards your spine, then move forward by moving your opposite hand and leg just 5–10 cm at a time. Move your right hand and left leg together, then your left hand and right leg.
- # Keep moving for up to 10 metres, but stop if you lose form before you get this far.
- # Once you can crawl forwards, try going backwards.

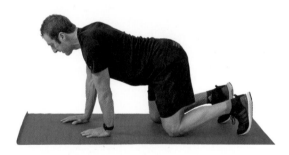

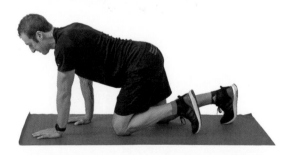

BEAR CRAWL

#· Crouch down, then place your hands on the ground so that they are directly under your shoulders. Straighten your arms and rise onto the balls of your feet. Your knees should not be on the ground.

Keeping your back in neutral, pull your belly button towards your spine, then crawl by moving your right hand and left foot forwards, followed by your left hand and right foot. Stay light on your hands and feet, and don't let your hips sit too high.

Once you have mastered the forward bear crawl, try going backwards, upstairs, uphill or downhill, or try it on the flat with some weight on your back.

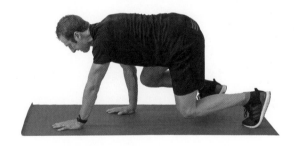

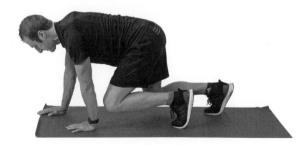

METABOLIC FINISHERS

To really hammer home the benefits of your workout, you can add a little extra!

Go stronger – Pick one of the previous exercises, and use a weight that is about 50–70% of the maximum that you can lift (so if you can lift 100 kg, use 70 kg). Then perform as many reps of your chosen exercise as you can, without losing form.

Go further – Jump on a rowing machine, bike, treadmill or use the stairs, park or track or an exercycle and go as far as you possibly can in 5 minutes. At each workout, try to increase the distance you go by 1%.

Go faster – On a treadmill set to a slight incline, or outside on an even surface, run as fast as you can for 30 seconds, then jog for 30 seconds. Repeat 5 times, for a total of 5 minutes.

NOW IT'S YOUR TURN

This might be the end of the book, but it's the beginning of your health journey. You know yourself – you've identified what good health means to you and why you want to achieve better health. You know your body – how your bones and muscles work, why some fat is good and some fat is bad, and how hormones and lack of sleep can drive you to donuts. You know what might get in the way of your goals – from friends and family to super-sizing and supermarkets.

You also know how to deal with all of these challenges, whether it's quieting the voice in your head, getting savvy with shopping strategies, or building bite-sized bits of exercise into your day.

Having this knowledge is one of the keys to your success. All that you have to do is apply it to your lifestyle. Look for those opportunities to tweak meals and activities and sleep habits so that you can take charge of your health. As well as the options suggested in this book there are bound to be many other tweaks that you can make. This is your life and you are the best person to know what you can achieve. The trick is to keep your eyes open for those opportunities, and then to act on them. Don't let inertia and apathy win the day – energy and enthusiasm are much better buddies to have on your side.

Remember, you don't have to make huge changes – a little will go a long way. Every time you add a healthy habit or quit an unhealthy one, you're creating a happier, healthier, fitter you – not just for today, but for the rest of your life.

It's over to you!

REFERENCES

CHAPTER 2

PAGE 14

1 in 3: Ministry of Health, Obesity Statistics. www.health.govt.nz/nz-health-statistics/health-statistics-and-data-sets/obesity-statistics

In 2014-2015: Ministry of Health, New Zealand Health Survey 2014/2015. www.health.govt.nz/publication/annual-update-key-results-2014-15-new-zealand-health-survey

Only one-third: Australian Institute of Health and Welfare, Overweight & Obesity. www.aihw.gov.au/who-is-overweight/

Obesity reduces: More Life, Consequences of Obesity. www.more-life.co.uk/Default.aspx?PageName=Consequences+of+Obesity

By 2016: World Health Organization, Obesity and Overweight. www.who.int/mediacentre/factsheets/fs311/en/

CHAPTER 8

PAGE 35

Choosing healthy food: University of Otago, Public Health Expert, 'Does healthy food really cost more?, Kate Sloane, posted 6 November 2014. blogs.otago.ac.nz/pubhealthexpert/2014/11/06/does-healthy-food-really-cost-more/

CHAPTER 9

PAGE 43

Our bones are living: Bart Clarke, Normal bone anatomy and physiology, Clin. J. Am. Soc. Nephrol, 2008, S131-S139, doi 10.2215/CJN.04151206. www.ncbi.nlm.nih.gov/pmc/articles/PMC3152283/

Like all living tissue: Osteoporosis Australia. www.osteoporosis.org.au/

PAGE 44

Get regular exposure: Ministry of Health, Vitamin D. www.health.govt.nz/your-health/healthy-living/food-and-physical-activity/healthy-eating/vitamin-d

PAGE 45

Rickets is a bone: O'Riordan, J & Bijvoet, O (2014), Rickets before the discovery of vitamin D, BoneKEy Reports, doi: 10.1038/bonekey.2013.212 www.nature.com/bonekeyreports/2014/140108/bonekey2013212/full/bonekey2013212.html?foxtrotcallback=true

The two bone-health: Bone Health and Osteoporosis: A report of the Surgeon-General. www.ncbi.nlm.nih.gov/books/NBK45503/

PAGE 46

The reason why men: Gkiatas, I, et al. (2015), Factors affecting bone growth, Am. J. Orthop. 44(1): 61-67

CHAPTER 10

PAGE 48

Just as your bones: Healthline, Testosterone levels by age. www.healthline. com/health/low-testosterone/testosterone-levels-by-age#adolescence3

At the gym: Dayanidhi, S & Lieber, R (2014) Skeletal muscle satellite cells: Mediators of muscle growth during development and implications for developmental disorders, Muscle Nerve, 50 (5): 723-732. doi: 10.1002/ mus.24441

PAGE 49

Say that instead: Holloszy, J & Coyle, E (1984) Adaptations of skeletal muscle to endurance exercise and their metabolic consequences, J. Appl. Physiol. 56 (4): 831-838. doi.org/10.1152/jappl.1984.56.4.831

CHAPTER 14

PAGE 106

Fat – now that's a word: Albright, A & Stern, J (1998) Adipose tissue. In: Encyclopedia of Sports Medicine and Science, T.D. Fahey (ed), Internet Society for Sports Science www.sportsci.org/encyc/adipose/adipose.html

White fat is regarded: University of Texas Health Centre at Houston (2013) New way to identify good fat, www.sciencedaily.com/ releases/2013/09/130918143311.htm See also: King, M (2017) Adipose tissue: not just fat, https://themedicalbiochemistrypage.org/adipose-tissue.php

PAGE 108

One thing that does: Lee, Y-H et al. (2014) Cellular origins of cold-induced brown adipocytes in adult mice, The FASEB Journal, doi.org/10.1096/fj.14-263038

So, we all have fat: Casey, J. Body fat measurement: percentage vs. body mass, www.webmd.com/diet/features/body-fat-measurement#2

PAGE 109

Exactly how visceral fat: Britten, K & Fox, C (2011) Ectopic fat depots and cardiovascular disease, Circulation (124): e837-e841. http://circ.ahajournals. org/content/124/24/e837

PAGE 111

OECD and obesity: OECD (2017) Obesity update, www.oecd.org/health/ obesity-update.htm

PAGE 112

If you wanted to: Jampolis, M (2011) Which test should I trust when measuring my body fat? http://edition.cnn.com/2011/HEALTH/expert.q.a/09/30/body.fat.testing.jampolis/index.html

PAGE 114

A survey of the world's 30: Maffetone, P, Rivera-Dominguez, I & Laursen, P (2017) Overfat adults and children in developed countries: the public health importance of identifying excess body fat, Front. Public Health http://journal.frontiersin.org/article/10.3389/fpubh.2017.00190/full

PAGE 115

Whether or not you: Strasser, B & Fuchs, D (2016) Diet versus exercise in weight loss and maintenance: focus on tryptophan, Int. J. Tryptophan Res. 9: 9-16 (biggest loser)

PAGE 116

If you need more convincing: Fothergill, E et al. (2016) Persistent metabolic adaptation 6 years after "The Biggest Loser" competition, Obesity 24 (8): 1612-1619 https://onlinelibrary.wiley.com/doi/full/10.1002/oby.21538

CHAPTER 15

PAGE 118

Insulin is a bit like: Insulin, effects. www.pharmacorama.com/en/Sections/Insulin_2.php

PAGE 120

Scientists have known: Tomiyama, A et al. (2010) Low calorie dieting increases cortisol, Psychosom. Med. 72 (4): 357-364. www.ncbi.nlm.nih.gov/pmc/articles/PMC2895000/

Cortisol has also: Aronson, D (2009) Cortisol – its role in stress, inflammation and indications for diet therapy, Today's Dietician, 11 (11): 38 www.todaysdietitian.com/newarchives/111609p38.shtml

PAGE 124

It's also important: Braatvedt, G et al. (2012) Understanding the new HbA1c units for the diagnosis of Type 2 diabetes, New Zealand Medical Journal, 125 (1362): 70-80. www.nzma.org.nz/journal/read-the-journal/all-issues/2010-2019/2012/vol-125-no-1362/article-braatvedt

Not only that: van Cauter, E et al. The impact of sleep deprivation on hormones and metabolism. www.medscape.org/viewarticle/502825

PAGE 125

A lot of people: Wilsmore, B et al. (2013) Sleep habits, insomnia, and daytime sleepiness in a large and healthy community-based sample of

New Zealanders, J. Clin. Sleep Med. 9 (6): 559-66. www.ncbi.nlm.nih.gov/pubmed/23772189

There are also: Howatson, G et al. (2012) Effect of tart cherry juice (Prunus cerasus) on melatonin levels and enhanced sleep quality, Eur. J. Nutr. 51 (8): 909-16. www.ncbi.nlm.nih.gov/pubmed/22038497. See also: Lin, H et al. (2011) Effect of kiwifruit consumption on sleep quality in adults with sleep problems, Asia Pac. J. Clin. Nutr. 20 (2): 169-74. www.ncbi.nlm.nih.gov/pubmed/21669584

CHAPTER 16

PAGE 132

Carbs and energy: Lovegrove, A et al. (2017) Role of polysaccharides in food, digestion and health, Crit. Rev. Food Sci. Nutr. 57 (2): 237-253. www.ncbi.nlm.nih.gov/pmc/articles/PMC5152545/

PAGE 134

Very recently, attention: PrecisionNutrition, Resistant starch: what is it ? And why is it so good for you? www.precisionnutrition.com/all-about-resistant-starch.

Resistant starch might: Whole Health Source, Butyric acid: an ancient controller of metabolism, inflammation and stress resistance? http://wholehealthsource.blogspot.co.nz/2009/12/butyric-acid-ancient-controller-of.html

PAGE 135

In New Zealand and Australia: Ministry of Health, Nutrient Reference Values for Australia and New Zealand, www.nrv.gov.au/nutrients/dietary-fibre. See also: University of Otago and Ministry of Health, 2011, A focus on nutrition: key findings of the 2008/09 New Zealand adult nutrition survey, Wellington, Ministry of Health

CHAPTER 17

PAGE 140

The protein story: The Open University, OpenLearn, www.open.edu/openlearn/science-maths-technology/science/biology/nutrition-proteins/content-section-1.7

PAGE 141

In developed countries: WebMD, Protein popularity: the evidence behind the hype. www.webmd.com/diet/news/20000425/protein-popularity#1

PAGE 142

The arrival of the Atkins: Wu, G (2016) Dietary protein intake and human health, Food Funct. 7 (3): 1251-65. www.ncbi.nlm.nih.gov/pubmed/26797090

CHAPTER 18

PAGE 144

The more the effects: Diabetes.co.uk, Low carb high fat diet. www.diabetes.co.uk/diet/low-carb-high-fat-diet.html

PAGE 147

Sleep smart: MedicalXpress (2017) Weekly fish consumption linked to better sleep, higher IQ, study finds. https://medicalxpress.com/news/2017-12-weekly-fish-consumption-linked-higher.html

PAGE 148

It's long been thought: Siri-Tarino P, Sun Q, Hu F, et al. (2010). Saturated fat, carbohydrate, and cardiovascular disease. The American Journal of Clinical Nutrition 91(3): 502-509.

The dietary omegas that: Weisenberger, J (2014) The omega fats, Today's Dietitian, 16 (4): 20. www.todaysdietitian.com/newarchives/040114p20.shtml

PAGE 151

Be careful with canola: MedicalXpress (2017) Canola oil linked to worsened memory and learning ability in Alzheimer's. https://medicalxpress.com/news/2017-12-canola-oil-linked-worsened-memory.html

PAGE 153

Will coconut fat make me thin?: Wosen, J (2017) How coconut oil got a reputation for being healthy in the first place. www.statnews.com/2017/06/20/coconut-oil-reputation-healthy/

CHAPTER 20

PAGE 160

You'll no doubt: Sawka, M, Cheuvront, S & Carter R (2005) Human water needs, Nutr. Rev. 63 (6): S30-9. www.ncbi.nlm.nih.gov/pubmed/16028570

PAGE 163

Drying out with alcohol: ABC Science, Why does drinking alcohol cause dehydration? www.abc.net.au/science/articles/2012/02/28/3441707.htm

PAGE 167

A few small studies: Mitrou, P et al. (2010) Vinegar decreases postprandial hyperglycemia in patients with Type 1 diabetes, Diabetes Care, 33 (2): e27. http://care.diabetesjournals.org/content/33/2/e27.full

A similar study: Johnston, C, Kim, C & Buller, A (2004) Vinegar improves insulin sensitivity to a high-carbohydrate meal in subjects with insulin resistance or Type 2 diabetes, Diabetes Care, 27 (1): 281-282. http://care.diabetesjournals.org/content/27/1/281

CHAPTER 23

PAGE 173

Green goodness: MedicalXpress (2017) One serving of leafy greens a day may slow brain aging by 11 years https://medicalxpress.com/news/2017-12-salad-day-memory-problems.html

CHAPTER 25

PAGE 179

And it's not just fast: Benton, D (2015) Portion size: what we know and what we need to know, Crit. Rev. Food Sci. Nutr., 55 (7): 988-1004. www.ncbi.nlm.nih.gov/pmc/articles/PMC4337741/#cit0111

PAGE 186

A tale of two diets: Portion sizes derived from information presented in Zheng, M et al. (2016) Typical food portion sizes consumed by Australian adults: results from the 2011-12 Australian National Nutrition and Physical Activity Survey, Sci. Rep. 6: 19596. www.ncbi.nlm.nih.gov/pmc/articles/PMC4726402/

CHAPTER 26

PAGE 194

Don't skip breakfast: MedicalXpress (2017) Skipping breakfast disrupts 'clock genes' that regulate body weight, https://medicalxpress.com/news/2017-11-breakfast-disrupts-clock-genes-body.html

PAGE 287

If you exercise: Asker Jeukendrup (2015) www.mysportscience.com/single-post/2015/04/30/Protein-intake-before-sleep-results-in-greater-muscle-mass-and-strength

PAGE 294

Your muscles burn energy: Moller, N and Nair, K (1999) Regulation of muscle mass and function: effects of aging and hormones. www.nap.edu/read/9620/chapter/10#122

INDEX

PENGUIN

UK | USA | Canada | Ireland | Australia
India | New Zealand | South Africa | China

Penguin is an imprint of the Penguin Random House group of companies, whose
addresses can be found at global.penguinrandomhouse.com.

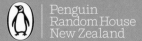

First published by Penguin Random House New Zealand, 2018

10 9 8 7 6 5 4 3 2 1

Design by Cat Taylor © Penguin Random House New Zealand
Prepress by Image Centre Group
Printed and bound in China through APOL, Hong Kong

A catalogue record for this book is available from the National Library of New Zealand.

ISBN 978-0-14-377211-8
eISBN 978-0-14-377212-5

The information contained in this book is of a general nature only. If you wish to
make use of any dietary or exercise information in this book relating to your health,
you should first consider its appropriateness to your personal situation, including
consulting a medical professional.

Back cover photograph © NewspixNZ/Andrew Warner; Getty Images: page 4 (Phil
Walter); pages 24–25 (Colin Anderson); iStock: pages 12–13 (Mutlu Kurtbas); page 21
(ozgurdonmaz); page 24 (Colin Anderson); pages 40–41, 82–83 (GlobalStock); pages
44, 56 (aydinmutlu); pages 47–48 (ninikas); pages 51, 85, 165 (Solovyova); pages
52–53 (MadamLead); pages 62–63 (Ivanko Brnjakovic); page 68 (egon69); page 72
(alffalff); page 79 (m-imagephotography); page 80 (Steevy84); page 89 (alvarez); page
127 (Vertigo3d); pages 128–129 (Lisovskaya); pages 138–139 (97); page 147 (alffalff);
page 151(Bozena Fulawka); page 153 (virtustudio); page 163 (mattjeacock); page 167
(virtustudio); page 170 (robynmac); page 176–177 (Denira777); page 181 (theJIPEN/
filistimlyanin); page 182 (Sitade); page 185 (baibaz); page 194 (Foxys forest manu-
facture); page 195 (Paul Maguire); pages 200–201 (Alex Raths); page 203 (Floortje);
pages 208–209 (OksanaKiian); pages 121–123 (Aleksandar Nakic); page 61(Steve
Debenport); page 64 (Nastasic); Shutterstock: page 134 (Piyaset): Wattbike image
(page 149) © Wattbike

penguin.co.nz

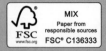